ANATOMIC PATHOLOGY FOR VETERINARY CLINICIANS

ANATOMIC PATHOLOGY FOR VETERINARY CLINICIANS

Melanie Dobromylskyj

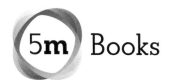

5m Books

First published 2023

Published by
5M Books Ltd
Lings, Great Easton
Essex CM6 2HH, UK,
Tel: +44 (0)330 1333 580
www.5mbooks.com

Follow us on
Twitter @5m_Books
Instagram 5m_books
Facebook @5mBooks
LinkedIn @5mbooks

A Catalogue record for this book is available from the British Library

ISBN 9781789182378
eISBN 9781789182453
DOI 10.52517/9781789182453

Book layout by Cheshire Typesetting Ltd, Cuddington, Cheshire
Printed by Hobbs the Printers
Photos by the author unless otherwise indicated

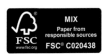

Contents

Abbreviations

ABC	avidin-biotin complex
ACVIM	American College of Veterinary Internal Medicine
AgNOR	argyrophilic nucleolar organizer regions
AL	amyloid light chain
AK	actinic keratosis
ARVC	arrhythmogenic right ventricular cardiomyopathy
BCR	B-cell receptor
DCM	dilated cardiomyopathy
DLBCL	diffuse large B-cell lymphoma
DNA	deoxyribonucleic acid
EATCL	enteropathy associated T-cell lymphoma
FIP	feline infectious peritonitis
FISH	fluorescence in situ hybridization
FISS	feline injection site sarcoma
GB	gigabyte
GFAP	glial fibrillary acidic protein
GI	gastrointestinal
GIST	gastrointestinal stromal tumour
GMS	Grocott's methenamine silver stain
HE	haematoxylin and eosin
HPF	high power field
HTFM	histological tumour free margins
HVG	haematoxylin van Gieson
IHC	immunohistochemistry
ISH	in situ hybridization
IVS	interventricular septum
KP	keratin pearls
LGAL	low grade alimentary lymphoma
LVFW	left ventricular free wall
MC	mitotic count
MCM	minichromosome maintenance

MCT	mast cell tumour
MF	mitotic figure
MHC	major histocompatibility complex
MMEE	mitotic-modified Elston-Ellis
MMM	masticatory muscle myositis
MSB	Martius scarlet blue
MST	median survival time
N:C	nuclear:cytoplasmic
PARR	PCR for antigen receptor rearrangements
PAS	periodic acid-Schiff
PCR	polymerase chain reaction
PME	postmortem examination
PTAH	Mallory's phosphotungstic acid haematoxylin
RBC	red blood cell
RNA	ribonucleic acid
RVFW	right ventricular free wall
SCC	squamous cell carcinoma
SMA	smooth muscle actin
STS	soft tissue sarcoma
TCR	T-cell receptor
TRH	thyrotropin releasing hormone
TSH	thyroid stimulating hormone
TTF1	thyroid transcription factor 1
TZL	T-zone lymphoma
UV	ultraviolet
VCGP	Veterinary Cancer Guidelines and Protocols
WHO	World Health Organization
WSAVA	World Small Animal Veterinary Association
ZN	Ziehl–Neelsen

Submission of samples

1

Introduction

This first chapter helps clinicians optimize their samples when submitting tissues to the laboratory for histopathological assessment; this includes both the submission form and the tissue sample itself. We will take a look at some clinical history 'dos and don'ts', some good and less good examples of sample packaging and at some of the issues that arise when samples are not fixed sufficiently, or are crushed, cauterized or otherwise mishandled. There will also be an overview of what happens to samples once they arrive at the laboratory, from trimming through to the final, often digitized, slides viewed by the reporting pathologist.

The submission form and the clinical history

One of the most important and often overlooked aspects of submitting laboratory samples for histopathology, and for other types of laboratory tests, is the submission form and the inclusion of vital information about the patient, the lesion and the pertinent clinical history. There is an old urban myth that when submitting a sample for analysis, you should not include a clinical history, or your clinical differential diagnoses, because you do not want to 'bias' the pathologist. Hopefully this chapter will help to debase that particular myth.

To perhaps put this into a more clinical-type setting, imagine that you are in a consultation but that you are not allowed to ask the owner any questions. Or maybe you are not allowed to physically examine the patient. Without these important sources of information, you are severely hampered in your ability to construct a meaningful working differential list, and the very same is true for pathologists too.

Not all clinical histories are equally good, however, and longer is not necessarily better.

A well completed submission form includes simple things like:

- including the signalment, with the species, breed, age, gender and, if relevant, the coat colour
- giving a brief but accurate summary of the clinical history:
  - onset and duration of any clinical signs
  - previous treatments and any response seen (or none)
  - description of any findings at exploratory surgery, imaging or post-mortem examination
- describing the lesion (see Chapter 2 for more on gross descriptions):
  - colour, size, texture, location and duration
  - increasing in size, or fluctuating
  - grown rapidly, or been present but slowly growing for a long time
  - changed in nature, become ulcerated or inflamed
  - fixed in place or mobile
  - pruritic or painful
- including any additional information:
  - is the biopsy excisional or incisional? Have you included margins for assessment?
  - if multiple samples are submitted, are they clearly labelled, and do they correspond to the submission form?
  - are any imaging results included?
  - are there any previous laboratory results?
- providing a list of your own differential diagnoses or clinical impressions and any specific questions which you have about the case.

What we do not really want with a submission are:

- blank forms, lacking even the practice name or address
- illegible handwriting
- a list of very obscure abbreviations which we struggle to decipher
- a 'copy and paste' of a part of the patient's clinical records, with the anaesthetic protocol, details of the surgical technique, the suture material used and the post-operative care plan, but no mention of the site or lesion itself (Figure 1.1)
- a print-out of the animal's entire history, as we often cannot find the relevant information among all of the practice management information, records of boosters and wormers, phone calls and messages left on the client's daughter's answerphone. (The current record holder for our laboratory is 156 pages, of which only the last 4 pages were relevant to the submission.)

MASS REMOVAL   GA-premed-medeto 0.02 and methadone 0.18ml. Induction with alfaxan. Intubated and maintenance with ISO/02. Eyelubed. IVFT 5ml/kg/hr. Elliptical incision around mass, subcut closed with monocryl 2M and skin closed with monocryl 2M. PLAN-*POC in 3 days, before if any worries. *keep ecollar on *rest and bland diet *gabapentin PO, starting tonight. *awaiting lab results. Dicharged by
Label: Dispensed 14 × Gabapentin Caps 100mg V.

Figure 1.1 Example of a 'copy and paste' clinical history, which neglects to include any information about the sample itself.

Sample packaging

Please do make use of appropriate sample containers, which should be screw-top and designed for the purpose of submitting histopathology samples. Try to avoid the temptation to get creative with margarine tubs, lunch boxes, glass coffee jars and various forms of Elastoplast, surgical or duct tape (Figure 1.2). Narrow-necked bottles in particular pose a significant problem; tissue samples will swell once placed in fixative and some will also become far less malleable. This means that samples that fitted nicely in through the neck of the bottle often will no longer fit out again once the sample arrives at the laboratory. This leads to us having to use saws and sometimes hammers (if containers are made of glass) to break into the container, potentially damaging the specimen and also putting laboratory staff at risk. For similar reasons, please do not leave sharp objects such as needles in samples.

Another classic improvised container is the sharps bin – but these are designed to not be reopened once sealed and again present us with a real challenge (Figure 1.3). Containers not designed for the purpose of submitting histopathology samples are also more likely to leak formalin, which is another hazard for anyone subsequently handling the submission.

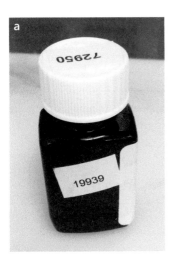
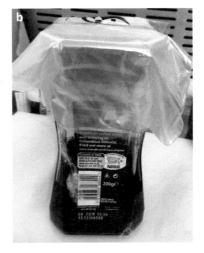
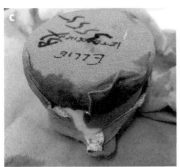
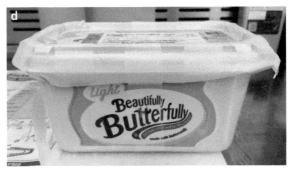

Figure 1.2 Inappropriate containers, for example, narrow-necked bottles, glass containers which are also not water-tight, containers encased in Elastoplast (which turns particularly gloopy and unpleasant when it comes into contact with formalin), or margarine tubs, no matter how 'beautifully butterfully'.

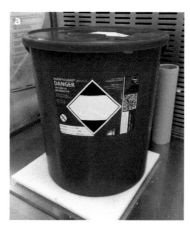
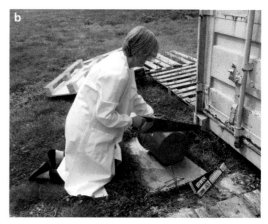

Figure 1.3 Sharps containers are specifically designed to not be re-openable once sealed, and so present us with a real challenge, including a risk to the health and safety of our staff. There is also a risk that we might damage the sample while trying to retrieve it from the container.

Labelling of sample pots, particularly if submitting more than one sample and from more than one site, is something which can be easily forgotten, but which can have dire consequences for the patient. If five masses are submitted from five different sites, and one is malignant, then it is vital that both the pathologist and the clinician can correlate those results back to the locations on the patient from which they came. Unfortunately, it sometimes happens that despite a perfectly detailed submission form, if the pots themselves are unlabelled it can be difficult or impossible to ascertain which mass came from where.

The importance of fixation

Using the correct amount and type of fixative is important. Ideally this should be a 10 : 1 volume ratio of formalin to tissue, and the formalin should be 10% neutral buffered formalin. Inadequate and/or delayed fixation can render a good sample completely non-diagnostic. Remember that formalin penetrates tissues at a relatively slow rate of approximately 1 mm per hour, and samples will fix from the outside in. This means that the central area of large specimens may not be fixed on receipt by the laboratory and will thus require further fixation before they can be processed. In the worst cases, samples received might be fixed on the outside, and putrid in the centre (Figure 1.4).

Using a sample container that is too small will not only result in inadequate fixation as too little formalin will be present, but it can also result in distortion of the sample. Samples such as this will swell and take on the shape of whatever container they were in, meaning that orientation of the specimen for trimming and margin assessment becomes difficult or sometimes impossible (Figure 1.5).

Trimming down of samples or serial slicing through organs, such as spleens, at 1 cm intervals will speed up the process of fixation by allowing better access of the formalin to these parts of the tissues. Overnight fixation for 1 cm thick slices of tissues is ideal. Please remember that adequate fixation should not be compromised in the interests of minimalizing turnaround times, and the length of time will vary depending on the sample size and type. Histopathology is a process that does take time, and although samples can be 'fast tracked' to some extent, the entire process from receiving a sample at the laboratory to the sample being trimmed into cassettes, the tissues processed, then embedded in wax, sectioned,

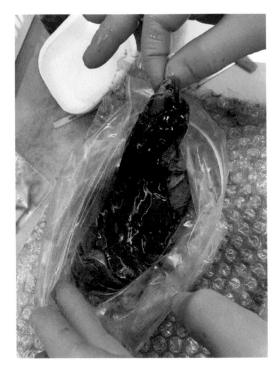

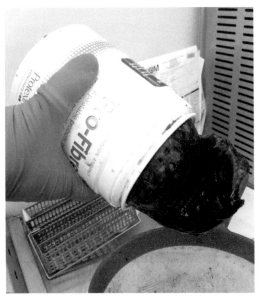

Figure 1.4 Example of an unfixed sample. This sample was submitted wrapped in formalin-soaked gauze but without prior fixation at the practice and unfortunately was non-diagnostic by the time it reached the laboratory.

Figure 1.5 This container is too small for the sample. There is insufficient space for an adequate volume of formalin, so tissue fixation is poor, the tissue has swollen, meaning the sample no longer fits through the narrow neck intact. The sample has also taken on the form of the pot, so inside the pot this spleen with an associated mass is now cylindrical in shape.

stained, dried and 'cover-slipped' on a slide before it reaches the pathologist to interpret does take a certain amount of time.

Submission of challenging samples

Submitting some types of samples for histopathology can be really challenging, for example mammary strips, amputated limbs, whole organs and very large tumours. This section gives some guidance for these difficult cases, but remember you can always speak to your laboratory first if you are unsure of what to do.

Larger tumours

Ask yourself the following questions.

1. Does the sample fit comfortably within one routine biopsy pot? Remember, please do not squeeze large samples into too small a pot.
   - Doing so will not allow for adequate fixation – the ideal tissue to formalin ratio should be 10 : 1; 5 : 1 or less is inadequate.

- The sample will take the form of the pot. Such samples are difficult or impossible to orient and to relate to the original specimen/in situ lesion, making accurate assessment of surgical margins in particular a real challenge.
- Please do not be tempted to use inappropriate containers to submit samples, and under no circumstances should a sharps bin, glass jar, Tupperware container or narrow-necked pot be used in replacement of a biopsy pot.

If the answer to question 1 is yes, follow the normal packaging guidelines for your laboratory. If no, progress to question 2.

2. Can the sample be cut in half and submitted in two pots? Or in quarters and into four pots? Please do not section into smaller proportions than quarters, as it becomes impractical to re-orient and process.

   If the answer to question 2 is yes:
   - Section the sample and submit in separate, clearly labelled biopsy pots.
   - These should be accompanied by a sketch or digital image of the original specimen to depict sectioning and orientation of the sample.
   - If margin evaluation is required, the surgical margins including the deep margin should be marked appropriately (for example, with surgical sutures or tissue ink, see Chapter 3 for more information).

   If no, move on to question 3.

3. Does the whole sample really need to be submitted?

   If the answer is no, then submit one (or more) relevant sections in one or more biopsy pots. Retain the remainder of the sample in fixative within the practice until the histopathology report is received – if the pathologist requires further tissues, these can then be submitted. Some samples are best submitted whole, for example, hearts, brains and sometimes spleens. If unsure, please speak to your laboratory first.

   If the answer to question 3 is yes, the whole sample does need to be submitted, then the sample will require fixation at the practice first prior to submission. It is important to ensure all local health and safety regulations are adhered to before you do this, and that your practice has suitable facilities for this to be done in a safe manner.

- First fix the sample in a large container with a lid at the practice, following local health and safety guidance.
- 10% neutral buffered formalin should be replaced with fresh solution after 24 hours if the specimen requires longer fixation.
- A ratio of less than 5 : 1 formalin : tissue is considered inadequate, optimal is 10 : 1.
- Consider slicing the sample, removing unnecessary muscle, fascia and so on to allow for penetration of formalin into the tissues – a series of partial incisions 1 cm apart into the centre of the tissue will aid tissue permeation and fixation.
- Consider de-bulking limbs of muscle and skin that will not be required for assessment.
- The length of time the samples should be left to fix at the surgery will depend on the size and type of tissue and method of transportation to the laboratory; formalin penetrates tissues very slowly at approximately 1 mm per hour, so specimens need to be left to fix for an adequate length of time.

- Specimens should be fixed for approximately 6–72 hours, preferably for a minimum of 8 hours or overnight, especially for larger specimens, at room temperature.
- Anatomical barriers to fixation should be removed or incised where possible (for example, fascia, bone, faeces, thick tissues); large samples should be sectioned or opened and gently cleaned (for example, gastrointestinal tract) to allow penetration of fixative. Remember not to scrape mucosal surfaces.
- Adequate fixation should not be compromised in the interests of minimalizing turnaround times.
- Once fixed, package as follows.
  - Wrap the sample in formalin-soaked gauze / tissue to keep the sample moist in transit.
  - Place inside two sealed leak-proof bags (clinical waste / cadaver bags recommended).
  - Wrap in absorbent material (newspaper / tissue).
  - Place inside a rigid container or box (please note a sharps bin is not a suitable container for this purpose).

Hearts

Submission of the whole heart, uncut, fixed in formalin is often the preferred sample, greatly increasing the likelihood of a diagnosis for conditions such as cardiomyopathy and congenital defects, as the pathologist can assess the gross specimen (Figure 1.6).

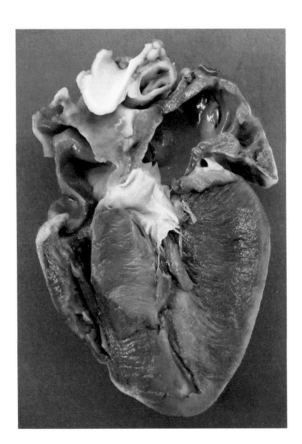

Figure 1.6 Fixed specimen, whole heart from a cat with cardiomyopathy, examined and sectioned by the pathologist.

- Remove the heart whole, and strip back the pericardium.
- Flush any blood and clots out from the chambers using water.
- Record the fresh weight of the heart (with any blood and clots flushed out of the chambers).
- Fix whole in formalin and submit.

Mammary tumours or strips

- Does the entire mammary strip need to be submitted, or is there a discrete mass of clinical concern? If the latter, then the mass and regional lymph nodes can be submitted separately; the remainder of the tissue can be retained in fixative in the practice until the final report is received.
- If necessary, the mass can be cut into sections and placed into individual labelled pots, and submitted with an accompanying trimming diagram or photographs as detailed above. Consider labelling of margins with ink or suture tags. Areas of interest/suspected masses should be clearly noted on the submission form/diagram.
- Some mammary masses may need to be cut with a saw if mineralized but hard portions need to be submitted as they are representative portions of the lesion. Some mammary samples may require chemical softening ('decalcification') once received by the laboratory and may have a longer turnaround time as a result.
- If the whole strip requires assessment, treat as a large sample, see above for further information.

Amputated limbs

- Does the whole limb need to be submitted? For example, if a bone tumour is suspected, then submit the portion of bone with the associated mass and bone for assessment in the first instance.
- Larger samples will take longer to fix and then to chemically soften, meaning a delayed report, possibly with poor tissue fixation hampering the histological assessment. Poor fixation and chemical softening will also greatly hamper any additional downstream testing such as immunohistochemistry.
- Consider de-bulking limbs of muscle and skin that will not be required for assessment.
- Retain the remainder of the sample, in formalin, in the practice until the final histopathology report is received.
- If examination of draining lymph nodes associated with limb amputations is required, the surgeon should consider dissecting the node and submitting it in a separate biopsy pot, as the lymph node can be difficult to identify following fixation if it is still within the limb tissue.
- If assessment of margins is required, these can also be submitted separately, either clearly marked for orientation, or as samples to determine the presence or absence of neoplastic tissue in the sample.

Spleens

Pathological changes within the spleen can generally be either diffuse or nodular in nature. Nodular lesions can be non-neoplastic or neoplastic, and either benign or highly malignant, and getting the diagnosis correct is critically important. However, often the lesion itself is obscured by extensive secondary, non-specific changes such as haemorrhage, congestion, haematoma formation and reactive fibroplasia, necrosis, extramedullary haematopoiesis and autolysis, and these changes can sometimes form the bulk of the mass seen grossly. Therefore, appropriate sample submission is crucial in trying to establish a correct diagnosis. Studies have found that the submission of the entire spleen is more likely to yield a definitive diagnosis than multiple sections.

If submitting the whole spleen, it is recommended to fix it initially at the practice before submitting it to the laboratory, as per the directions above. A series of partial incisions should be made through the capsule at approximately 1 cm intervals to allow better penetration of formalin and more rapid fixation of the deeper tissues. If it is not possible to submit the whole spleen, then selective sampling of the affected portions of the spleen followed by fixation will help to improve the diagnostic rate. Try to select slices of tissue that incorporate different areas of change and that span the periphery of the lesion and the surrounding 'normal' splenic tissues, in a radial fashion around any masses present. Also sample and submit any areas of adhesion or extra-splenic omental lesions, as well as any lymph nodes which may be enlarged. Keep the remaining tissue fixed at the clinic until the final histopathology report is received, in case any additional material is requested. Do remember however, that a diagnosis cannot always be achieved in every case, despite numerous sections being taken and examined, due to the extensive secondary changes sometimes present, which may obscure the primary pathology.

Tissue handling and artefacts

Tissue handling is crucial; think about which tissues you will be submitting for histopathology, including the margins, and try not to handle those areas more than is necessary, to avoid crushing the tissues that the histopathologist will need to assess (Figure 1.7).

The following should be avoided if at all possible.

- Avoid crushing the sample. Crush artefact means that the tissues can become distorted and cells become unrecognizable, the surgical margins can be impossible to assess, and if the crushing is severe enough unfortunately it can render the sample non-diagnostic (Figure 1.8).
- Avoid cauterizing the sample itself. Cautery heats the tissues and essentially cooks it. This can result in the loss of most of the tissue detail, particularly the margins, but if the sample is small then all of the tissue might be adversely affected (Figure 1.9).
- Avoid scraping mucosal surfaces such as the gastrointestinal tract – this will most likely also remove the mucosa, which is probably the most important part. If the gastrointestinal contents really need to be removed, consider rinsing gently with water before fixation. Blood clots, for example in a heart, can also be gently flushed out prior to fixing.
- Please do not leave tissue samples sitting around – it is best to fix them straight away, ideally within 30 minutes. Tissues will start to degenerate very quickly, including those such as the pancreas and any mucosal surfaces, more so at high ambient temperatures.
- Please do not freeze the sample – freeze and thaw results in marked tissue artefacts and loss of much of the cellular and nuclear detail. It will also adversely affect techniques such as immunohistochemistry. If in doubt, it is best to cool a sample in a refrigerator while making further decisions.

- Do not package cytology and histopathology samples together – the formalin fumes will cause severe artefacts in the cytology samples and render them largely uninterpretable. Always package these types of samples separately.

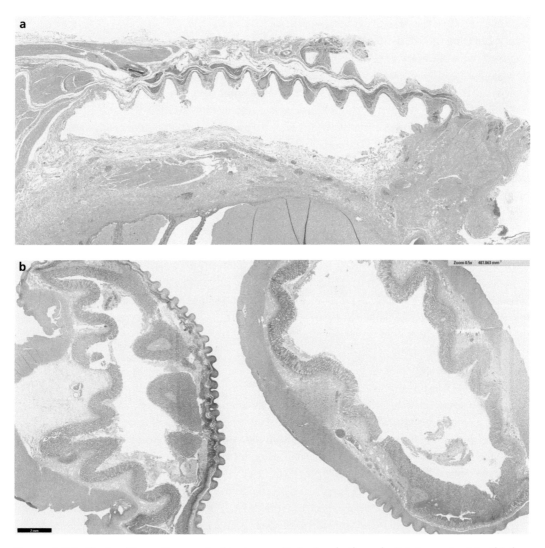

Figure 1.7 Let's play 'Guess the surgical instrument'. Seriously though, it is important to think about tissue handling when sampling for histopathology. Try to avoid handling the tissue to be submitted if possible. If the pathologist can identify which surgical instrument you were using to take the sample, this is probably not a good thing.

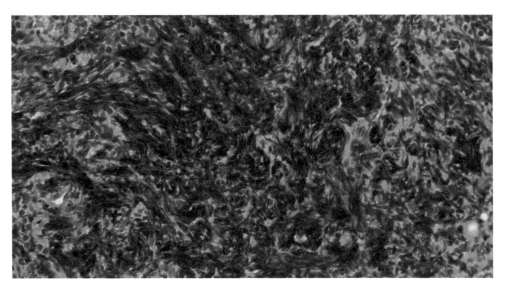

Figure 1.8 Crush artefact, in this case with nuclear streaming resulting in loss of nuclear detail, including nuclear morphology, whether the cell population is mixed, the degree of anisokaryosis and whether there is any evidence of mitotic activity.

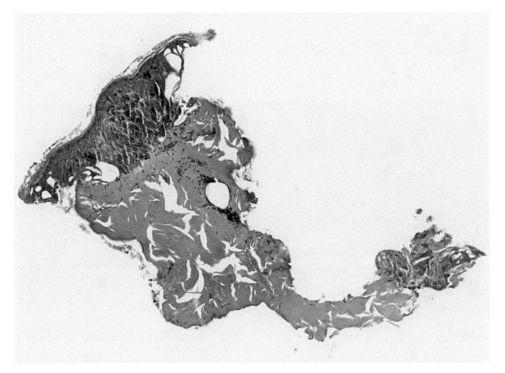

Figure 1.9 Cauterization of samples, which cooks the tissue and results in the loss of most of the tissue detail, particularly if the sample is small. This was a sample from an oral mass.

What happens to a sample when it reaches the lab?

This section describes what happens to the histopathology sample once it arrives at the laboratory, from receipt through to the report which is issued to you.

1 Sample reception

Samples are received in a reception area, where they are carefully unpackaged, checked and triaged towards the relevant laboratory department(s) for the requested testing (Figure 1.10) Details will be booked into a computer system, and a case number generated. Samples will be labelled and then transported to histology laboratory. A support team member may well contact the practice with any queries arising from the submission, for example an absent clinical history.

2 Histology laboratory

Once received in the histology laboratory, the tissue samples undergo a number of processing steps.

2.1 Fixation

To prevent autolysis and decay, and to preserve cells and tissues, samples will have been undergoing a process called fixation, starting at the practice as soon as the sample is placed in formalin, continuing during transportation to the laboratory and if necessary for a further period after receipt of the sample at the laboratory. Fixation stops enzyme activity within the tissues, kills any microorganisms present, and hardens the tissue specimen while maintaining the tissue architecture itself intact. The fixing agent is formaldehyde, usually in the form of a phosphate-buffered solution (referred to as formalin). Ideally, specimens should be fixed by immersion in formalin for 6 to 12 hours before they are processed, depending on their size.

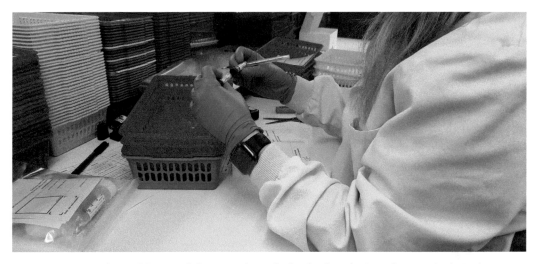

Figure 1.10 Samples will be carefully unpackaged, checked and triaged towards the relevant laboratory department(s) for the requested testing upon their receipt.

2.2 Trimming

Specially trained technicians will examine the specimen, noting the appearance, numbers of samples, size and so on, and may draw annotated diagrams to help the pathologist relate the sections on their slides to the sample received (Figure 1.11). Some more complex specimens require a pathologist to assist or trim the samples themselves. Larger specimens require dissection to produce representative sections from appropriate areas that fit into the tissue cassettes; smaller samples are most often processed whole.

Note that a tissue cassette typically measures only 3 × 2.5 × 0.4 cm so sections have to be smaller than this (Figure 1.12). Batches of tissue cassettes are loaded onto a tissue processor for processing through to wax.

2.3 Processing

Automated machines called tissue processors (Figure 1.13) are used to process large numbers of tissue samples – these machines pass the tissues through a sequence of different solvents: the tissue specimens are in an aqueous environment to start with and must be passed through multiple changes of dehydrating and clearing solvents (typically ethanol and xylene) before they can be placed in molten wax (which is hydrophobic and immiscible with water).

The duration and steps of the processing programme used will depend somewhat on the nature and size of the specimens, and often the bulk of processing is carried out overnight. Some laboratories may offer a fast-track service with a more rapid processing schedule for urgent cases, but please note that certain tissues are not suitable for this treatment (fatty, poorly fixed, bloody or lymphoid rich tissues in particular). Rapid processing such as this often results in sections of reduced quality, and also has potential to impact on downstream testing such as immunohistochemistry, which is why it tends not to be used for routine samples despite the theoretical advantage of a shorter turnaround time.

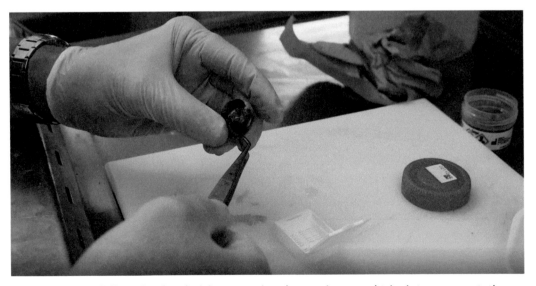

Figure 1.11 Specially trained technicians examine the specimen and trim into representative sections to fit into tissue cassettes.

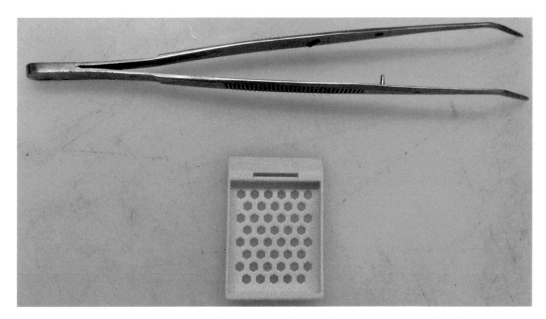

Figure 1.12 A tissue cassette into which sections of a sample must be trimmed to fit.

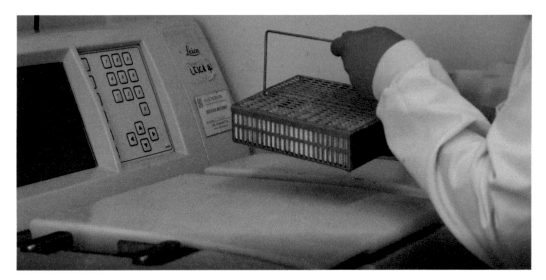

Figure 1.13 An automated tissue processing machine being loaded with tissue cassettes, processing samples to a stage where they can be immersed in molten wax.

2.4 Embedding

After processing, the specimens are placed in an embedding centre where they are removed from their cassettes and placed in wax-filled moulds (Figure 1.14). At this stage, specimens are carefully orientated because this determines the plane through which the section will be cut to ensure the areas of interest will be visible on the slide. The cassette in which the tissue has been processed

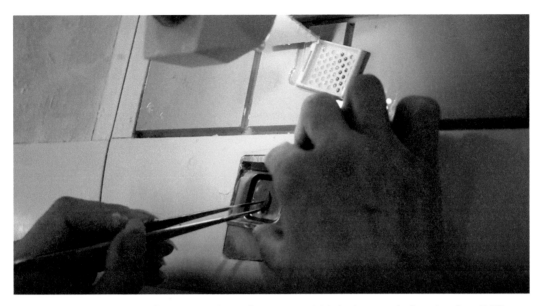

Figure 1.14 Embedding of specimens in molten wax, which is then cooled so that it solidifies to form a solid block of wax containing the tissue.

carries the identifying case and section number and is placed on top of the mould and attached by adding further wax. The wax containing the specimen is left to solidify on a cold surface, and when set, the mould is removed to leave a block of wax containing the tissue. The plastic tissue cassette forms part of this block, allowing identification and providing a base for clamping into the microtome.

2.5 Sectioning

Sections are cut on a microtome using extremely fine steel blades. Paraffin sections are usually cut at a thickness of 4–5 μm, depending on the laboratory, ensuring that only a single layer of cells makes up the section. As the sections are cut, they stick together edge-to-edge, forming a 'ribbon' of sections (Figure 1.15). Sections are 'floated out' on the surface of warm water in a water bath and picked up onto microscope slides. They dry and then they are ready to stain.

2.6 Staining and cover-slipping

Most of the cells and tissues are colour-less (except for pigments such as melanin), therefore sections have to be stained before they can be viewed. The routine stain is the haematoxylin and eosin (HE) stain, which stains cell nuclei blue, and cytoplasm and many extra-cellular components in varying shades of pink. Occasionally special stains are needed for other pigments or organisms, which may by requested by the pathologist after having first assessed the HE slides. Staining may be performed using an automated stainer, but more specialized stains may be applied by hand (Figure 1.16). After staining, the sections are covered with a coverslip.

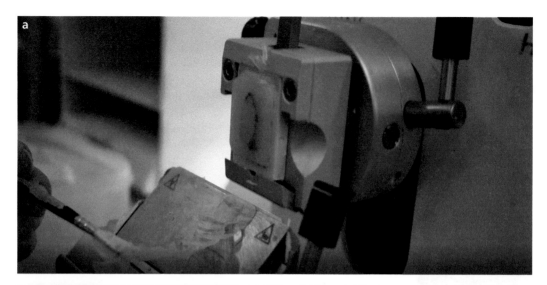

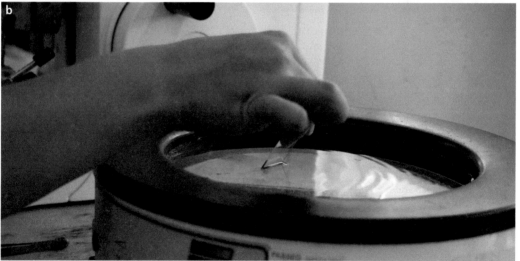

Figure 1.15 Sections are cut on a microtome and 'floated out' on warm water in a water bath, before being picked up onto microscope slides.

2.7 Quality check

Glass slides are labelled. The wax blocks and glass slides are checked against each other and against the submission form and trimming notes for any inconsistencies, and the slides are checked for any obvious quality issues.

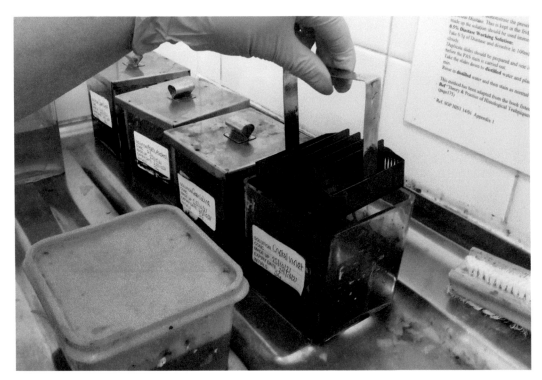

Figure 1.16 Some staining of sections may be done by hand, particularly some of the more specialized stains.

3 Digitization

Many diagnostic laboratories now operate digitally, which involves scanning the glass slides to produce a digital image, which the pathologist then views via a computer screen rather than assessing the glass slide down a conventional microscope. This process involves additional steps; the team receives the slides from the histology laboratory and are often responsible for scanning the slides and allocating cases to the relevant pathologists. They must first carefully clean and check the glass slides, as any debris can contaminate the digital scanner and cause harm to the machines.

These machines are capable of scanning at high resolution – typically they can scan at a resolution equivalent to the 400 × high-power lens on a microscope, and produce digital images that are then uploaded onto a server. The amount of time taken to scan a particular slide depends on the area of tissue present, but typically a slide takes approximately 1 minute to scan.

4 The histopathologist

The digital images of the scanned slides are viewed by pathologists, either working on-site or at locations remote to the laboratory (Figure 1.17). Pathologists access the digital images using a viewing platform and assess the slides, requesting any additional sections or special stains if required. Pathologists then compose and issue the report that makes its way to you.

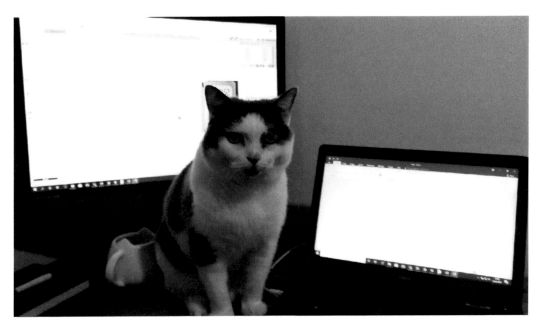

Figure 1.17 Working from home has its pros and cons.

Self-assessment: multiple choice questions

1. A Great Dane has undergone limb amputation surgery for a suspected bone tumour affecting the distal femur. You want to submit the sample for histological assessment, but is far too large for any of the routine sample pots. Which of the following should you do?
   a   Wrap the sample in formalin-soaked gauze to keep it moist in transit and submit it straight away before it undergoes autolysis.
   b   Ensure all of the skin, muscle, lymph nodes and marginal tissues are kept together, as it is vital that all of it is submitted for assessment in one piece.
   c   Remove normal tissues like muscle and skin, cut down the sample to the portion of bone with the lesion and place in fixative as soon as possible.
   d   Ensure there is a 5:1 formalin:tissue ratio so that the sample will fix nice and slowly.
2. Sample containers should be:
   a   easily breakable so that the sample can be retrieved by the laboratory personnel
   b   screw-top, water-tight and designed for the purpose of submitting samples for histopathology
   c   re-enforced with surgical or duct tape in case of formalin leakage during transit
   d   small enough that the sample will be held snugly in place during transit, to avoid damaging the sample.
3. What details DO NOT need to be on a sample submission form?
   a   The animal's age.
   b   The practice details.

   c The owner's phone number.

   d Where the sample was taken from.

4. You should never package cytology and histopathology samples together because:

   a the laboratory might get them muddled up and perform the wrong test on the wrong sample

   b if one sample gets lost in transit, you should still have the second sample

   c the formalin fumes will make the labels come off

   d the formalin fumes will affect the cytology samples.

5. Crush artefact can result in what changes in the tissues:

   a nuclear streaming, with loss of nuclear detail

   b the tissue to swell in size and become less malleable

   c damage of the tissues due to heat

   d loss of the mucosal layer.

The answers are available on page 167.

Self-assessment: case study

Case background

The patient is a 10-year-old, female (neutered) domestic short hair cat named Poppy, belonging to a Mr and Mrs Doolittle. Poppy initially presented to you a fortnight ago, when she had a palpable but rather indistinct, subcutaneous swelling over the inner aspect of the upper left forelimb. Today the physical examination suggests it is extending to involve the ventral thorax on that side. The area is dark pink to red and warm to the touch, and she rather resents you palpating it. The axillary and pre-scapular lymph nodes feel slightly enlarged on the left side when compared to the right. Physical examination does not reveal any other lymphadenopathy or lesions, and she is not pyrexic or otherwise systemically unwell. She has now been treated with antibiotics for 2 weeks without any obvious sign of improvement. A previous cytology sample came back as inflammatory, but with no evidence of infectious agents. You decide further investigation is warranted and that you wish to submit further samples to the laboratory.

    Please answer the following questions.

1. What are your differential diagnoses?

2. What samples would you submit and how would you preserve these?

3. What contact information needs to be included on the form?

4. What information is required about the owner and animal?

5. Can you prove a clinical summary – maximum 200 words?

6. Is there any other extra information you would like to include?

The answers are available on page 168.

Post-mortem examinations and gross pathology

2

Introduction

This chapter provides a detailed protocol for performing a thorough post-mortem examination in a small animal practice setting, together with details of the type of equipment required and information on collecting the best samples for further tests, such as histopathology, microbiology and toxicology. It also covers some areas to consider before embarking on the process itself – obtaining the relevant history, health and safety considerations, and note-taking. Remember that not all post-mortem examinations will result in a definitive diagnosis, and in many cases further tests such as histopathology will still be required; owners should be made aware of this. There is also a short section on how to 'gross' lesions, applicable to not just post-mortem settings but to any instance when the clinician needs to convey to the pathologist how a particular lesion appeared.

Performing a small animal post-mortem examination

Performing a really thorough post-mortem in practice is possible but it does require adequate time, a systematic and consistent approach and the right equipment (see Box 2.1). There are several possible reasons why a post-mortem might be requested. One of the most common is an apparently sudden or unexplained death, but other reasons include to confirm or refine a clinical diagnosis, to obtain samples for further tests (microbial culture, histopathology), to assess the effect of treatment(s), to collect evidence in forensic cases, or to prevent further illnesses and deaths among in-contact animals, for example, arising within litters of young puppies or kittens.

Box 2.1 **Post-mortem equipment checklist**

Post-mortem knife
Scissors (sharp and blunt ended)
Rat tooth forceps
Scalpel blade plus holder
Sample pots, empty and with formalin
Microbial swabs
Camera
Ruler
Note-taking equipment
Personal protective equipment
Cutting boards
Bone cutters, T-piece, saw
Scales
Syringes, measuring cylinder
Glass slides, coverslips, tape and appropriate stains for cytology samples and wet preparations

There are several important things to consider before you start. It is critical to obtain informed consent from the owner, and this should be accompanied by a signed consent form. The owners should be aware of what will happen to any samples taken during the process, and importantly that they will be unable to take the animal's remains home – ahead of the procedure, provision for alternative arrangements should be made, such as individual cremation with return of ashes. It is also important to have a full clinical history, including signalment, underlying conditions, clinical signs and current treatments, when and where the death occurred, and how: via euthanasia, unwitnessed or accompanied by signs such as seizuring. It is also useful to know how and for how long the body has been stored prior to post-mortem; remember that freeze–thaw artefacts will severely affect the quality of any tissue samples taken for histopathology, so it is best to avoid if possible.

Remember to consider the health and safety implications to both yourself and other staff and animals within the practice. Basic personal protective equipment should include disposable gloves and aprons and ideally cut-proof gloves. If there is any indication of zoonotic or highly infectious disease, then the case must be dealt with somewhere with the appropriate containment facilities. It may also be appropriate for certain cases to be dealt with by a professional veterinary pathologist, particularly if there are legal implications. Examples include forensic cases, potential welfare cases or if there is any question that the cause of death may be related to management of the case; referral of such cases to a specialist pathology service such as provided by a veterinary school is advisable. This is partly to ensure continuity of evidence, which is required if the post-mortem findings are to be used subsequently as evidence in court. The person performing the post-mortem may also be required to attend court proceedings and act as an expert witness.

The examination should be performed on a raised table in a well-lit room. Please bear in mind that post-mortems are dirty procedures and should be undertaken in an area where there is adequate drainage, and where thorough cleaning and disinfection are possible. The time required for such cleaning also needs to be considered and for these reasons, larger animals may be best referred to a specialist pathology service.

Assistance from a veterinary nurse or undergraduate veterinary student is extremely helpful for note-taking and photography. Note-taking is important: describe your gross findings and record them on submission forms accompanying samples for further testing. Most laboratories are also happy to receive digital photographs, which can be very useful – remember to include some indication of scale, such as a ruler, in each photo. Consider recording weights of organs, such as the thymus, or any organs which seem larger or smaller than expected.

External examination

Start by weighing the animal, removing and recording any collars, bandages or other materials, checking for any microchips and noting the body condition score. Record whether *rigor* (Latin, 'stiffness') and/or *algor mortis* (Latin, 'coldness') is present – this combination is particularly helpful in assessing the time from death, that is, the sequence is warm flaccid carcass, warm stiff carcass, cold stiff carcass then cold flaccid carcass. Note the extent of any post-mortem changes. Carefully examine all external structures and surfaces including the hair coat (note any clipped or alopecic areas, venipuncture sites), skin (for example, evidence of petechiae, bruising, icterus, oedema, lesions, tattoos, cutaneous tumours, scars, or other identifying markers), mucous membranes (for example, pallor, icterus, petechiae), eyes (including any discharge) and orifices (nares, ears, mouth including teeth, tongue and pharynx, anus, urogenital – discharges, faecal staining). Note any bony malformations, fractures or palpable masses. In some cases, such as those with potential trauma, bone pathology, or where there are forensic considerations, radiographs or other forms of imaging may be obtained prior to commencing the post-mortem examination. Examine the feet, and the nails for evidence of scuffing.

Opening the body cavities

Place the animal on its back. Make deep incisions in both axillae between the thoracic wall and the forelimbs (see Figure 2.1, incision 1) – reflect the forelimbs away from the body wall and lay them flat to stabilize the body in steady dorsal recumbence (see Figure 2.2, incision 1). Reflect the pelvic limbs in a similar way, by dissecting open the hip joints and laying the pelvic limbs out flat (Figures 2.1 and 2.2, incision 1).

Make a ventral midline incision through the skin from the mandibular symphysis to the pubis (Figure 2.2, incision 2). Reflect the skin back from the incision by cutting through the subcutaneous fat (Figure 2.2, incision 3); note the amount and colour of the subcutaneous adipose tissue – is there any evidence of oedema or bruising?

Slice through, examine and collect any superficial lymph nodes required, for example, the pre-scapular lymph nodes; you should be able to see distinct cortical and medullary zones within the lymph nodes. Peripheral lymph nodes can be difficult to locate unless enlarged, particularly in an animal with abundant subcutaneous fat – if you cannot find them, it probably means they are not significantly enlarged.

To expose the abdominal viscera, make a full incision through the ventral midline from the xiphoid process to the pubis – the linea alba should be elevated from the abdominal contents when making the midline incision to avoid inadvertent puncture of the abdominal viscera – particular care is needed here if there is post-mortem decomposition and gas accumulation. Extend the incision through the left and right sides of the abdominal wall caudal to the diaphragm and costal arch (Figures 2.3 and 2.4).

Be careful not to puncture the thoracic cavity. Examine the abdominal viscera in situ and check they are intact, the right size and in the right location – make a note of any abnormal fluid present in the abdomen, giving an approximate volume, colour, consistency and clarity (take a sample if the fluid appears

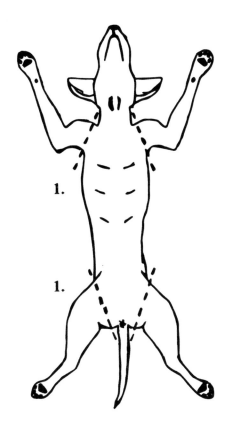

Figure 2.1 Place the animal on its back and stabilize the body by making incisions in both axillae and both hip joints (incision 1).

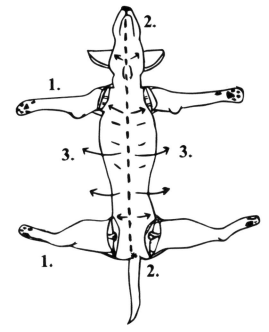

Figure 2.2 Reflect the forelimbs and the hind limbs away from the body wall and lay them flat to stabilize the body in a steady position. Make a ventral midline incision through the skin from the mandibular symphysis to the pubis (incision 2). Reflect the skin back from the incision by cutting through the subcutaneous fat (incision 3, arrows).

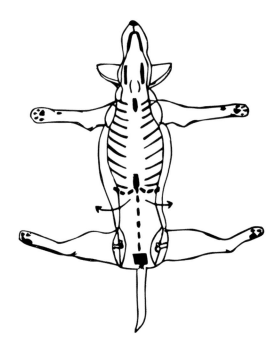

Figure 2.3 Make a full incision through the ventral midline from the xiphoid process to the pubis into the abdominal cavity. Extend the incision along the posterior margin of the last ribs on both sides and fold out the abdominal wall to expose the abdominal viscera in situ (arrows).

abnormal). Next, watch closely as you make a small stab incision through the diaphragm and verify the presence of negative pressure in the thorax by observing and listening for the influx of air – you should see the diaphragm move towards the abdominal cavity and become less tense. Cut a line through the soft tissues down to the bone along both sides of the ribcage. Using bone-cutters, cut through each rib

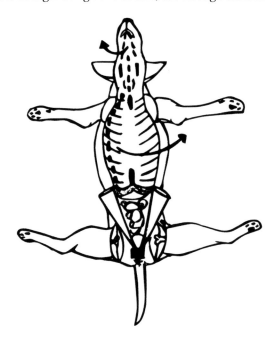

Figure 2.4 Cut a line through the soft tissues down to the bone and then using bone-cutters, cut through each rib along one side. Reflect the sternum and the attached portions of ribs over to reveal the thoracic viscera in situ (arrow). Incise through the soft tissues between the mandibles through to the oral cavity and pull the tongue through the floor of the mouth (arrow).

along one side (Figure 2.4) – you should now be able to reflect the sternum and the attached portions of ribs over to reveal the thoracic viscera in situ.

You should then be able to use a knife to just cut through the opposite site of the thoracic wall at the level of the costochondral junction – these joints normally break at this point meaning bone-cutters are not required for the second side. As with the abdomen, check for any fluid present within the thorax (take a sample if indicated) and for any displacement of organs.

Thorax

Start by incising the soft tissues between the mandibles through to the oral cavity and pulling the tongue through the floor of the mouth (Figure 2.4). Applying gentle traction on the tongue, continue to free the tongue, oropharynx and larynx from surrounding connective tissues. Incise across the soft palate, through the joints in the hyoid apparatus (these can be tricky!) and continue to dissect the connective tissues to remove the oesophagus, trachea, lungs and heart out as one (termed the pluck) – you will need to cut through the oesophagus, caudal vena cava and aorta at the level of the diaphragm to finally free the pluck from the thoracic cavity. Do not forget to check the tonsils, retropharyngeal and other regional lymph nodes and the salivary glands.

Once the pluck is removed, place it on a separate board or table. Identify and remove the thyroid and parathyroid glands. Remember if this is a young animal to check and remove the thymus. Open the oesophagus along the entire length, examine the internal surface and note any contents. Open the trachea from the larynx to the primary bronchi; again, note the internal surface and any contents. Palpate all the lung lobes and note any external lesions, areas of consolidation or haemorrhage and their pattern of distribution. Check the bronchial lymph nodes too for any enlargement or discoloration. Open along all the major bronchi into the lung parenchyma, again noting any contents; take a swab for microbial culture if respiratory disease is suspected. Collect tissue samples for histology from several of the lung lobes, ensuring a good section through the lung including major and minor airways through to the pleural surface. It is also good to note if the pieces of lung float in formalin, as this means they contain air rather than something more solid. Slice through the remaining lung parenchyma in parallel cuts at approximately 1 cm intervals, like slicing a loaf of bread, and examine the cut surfaces.

Heart

Next examine the heart, great vessels and pericardial sac in situ; incise the pericardial sac and note any abnormalities of the pericardial fluid. Reflect the sac up over the base of the heart and examine the base of the heart for any external masses or irregularities. Examine the great vessels and atria, epicardial surface and coronary vessels. Dissect the heart away from the remaining pluck, wash gently in water to remove as much blood as possible from within the cardiac chambers and obtain a weight – the normal weight for most animals is up to 1% of body weight, with exceptions for very young, athletic or cachexic animals.

The whole heart can be fixed in formalin – for cats this can be in a normal sample pot, but for larger canine hearts it may initially need fixing in a large volume of formalin in the practice before submission. This is often the preferred sample if submitted uncut and fixed, as the pathologist can then undertake a thorough assessment of the gross specimen before trimming. There are different approaches taken to sectioning hearts, depending on the pathologist; one traditional approach is the 'inflow–outflow method',

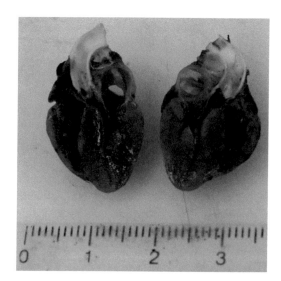

Figure 2.5 A very small kitten heart, opened
using the 5-chamber view.

but an alternative approach is one which mirrors the 4-chamber and 5-chamber views seen on echocardiography (Figure 2.5).

The 'inflow–outflow' method

Identify the right side of the heart and make an incision into the right atrium and then down through the right atrioventricular valve into the right ventricle, just to the edge of the coronary groove. To open the left side, make an incision directly through the middle of the ventricle starting from the atrium and extending to the apex, cutting through the left atrioventricular valve. Rinse the endocardial surface thoroughly and examine the endocardium, looking for areas of pallor, depressions, thickening or discoloration, and the atrioventricular valves looking for any nodules, misshaped or thickening of the valve leaflets. Check for any evidence of atrial or ventricular septal defects. Cut up into the great vessels and examine the aortic and pulmonary valves. Examine the myocardium on cut surfaces.

The 5-chamber approach

The 5-chamber approach, adopted from Dr Phil Fox, is particularly useful for cases with suspected left-sided disease and the vast majority of feline cases. This is a longitudinal section from base to apex, cutting through the aortic root and mitral annulus. Place the fixed heart vertically. Palpate the mitral annulus, make a stab incision into the left atrium and insert probe/forceps through the left atrium into the left ventricle. Dissect along the aorta until you reach the annulus, then insert a second probe/forceps down the left ventricular outflow tract into the left ventricle. Align the two pairs of forceps, place the blade between the prongs of both sets of forceps, and transect the heart with one cut downwards from base to apex, with the blade directed though the aortic root and mitral annulus simultaneously.

Dr Philip Fox is a specialist in veterinary cardiology, based at the Schwarzman Animal Medical Center, New York. He has published extensively within this field and a co-author of the recent ACVIM consensus statement guidelines for the classification, diagnosis, and management of cardiomyopathies in cats (Luis Fuente et al., 2020).

The 4-chamber approach

The 4-chamber approach, also from Dr Phil Fox, should be used in cases with suspected right-sided disease, most dogs and cats with suspected arrhythmogenic right ventricular cardiomyopathy (ARVC) or dilated cardiomyopathy (DCM). This technique is very similar to the 5-chamber view above, except that the second set of forceps are placed through the right atrium, right atrioventricular valve and into the right ventricle.

Whichever technique is used, it is important to ensure all parts of the heart are assessed, including external surface, great vessels, myocardium, endocardium and all valves. Measure the thickness of the right ventricular free wall, interventricular septum and the left ventricular free wall (the normal ratio is approximately 1 : 3 : 3 for the right ventricular free wall: interventricular septum: left ventricular free wall); this should be perpendicular to the long axis at approximately one-third of the way up from the apex, but do not take your measurements through the papillary muscles.

Abdominal contents

Locate both adrenal glands. Locate the cranial pole of the kidney, adjacent to renal blood vessels (Figure 2.6), examine the cut surfaces and collect in formalin. Make a small incision into the duodenum and then verify the patency of the bile duct by gently applying pressure to the gall bladder while observing for bile expulsion in the duodenum. Remove the spleen by cutting along the mesentery; place it on a separate board or table. Check the pancreas, both limbs. Straighten out the intestines by dissecting through the mesentery, cutting along the mesenteric attachments. Then cut the stomach free from the oesophagus and cut through the rectum; remove the gastrointestinal tract from the abdomen. Cut the liver and gall bladder out of the abdomen and place them on a separate board or table. Once removed from the abdominal cavity, examine the spleen and serially section, like the loaf of bread again. Open and examine the gall bladder, noting the amount, colour and consistency of the contents. Examine the surface of the liver lobes, noting any lesions or masses, the colour (or patterns of colours), size and consistency of the liver (for example, fatty, firm, nodular). Serially section the liver and examine the cut surfaces.

Examine the iliac lymph nodes and abdominal aorta in situ, by opening to the bifurcation. Free both kidneys from their attachments, bluntly dissect the ureters and urinary bladder and incise through the urethra. Once removed, incise and reflect the renal capsules to the hilus (Figure 2.7). Section both kidneys to the renal pelvis, cutting longitudinally (do not hold the kidneys in your hand when cutting – place them on a board). Note if ovariohysterectomy or castration have occurred, and if applicable check the location and number of testes. Note the contents of the urinary bladder and open to examine internal surface. Open the urethra, check the prostate gland (if applicable). For entire males, section the testes longitudinally. For entire females, remove the ovaries and uterus and incise to check internal surfaces of the genital tract.

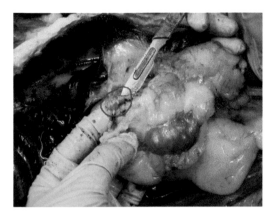

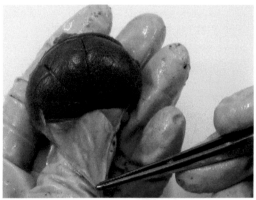

Figure 2.6 Locating the adrenal glands: this can be difficult as they may be deeply embedded in perirenal fat. Look at the cranial pole of the kidney, adjacent to renal blood vessels. Locating the adrenal glands is one of the first things I do on opening the abdomen, before they get 'lost' as other organs are moved about.

Figure 2.7 Incise and reflect the renal capsules to the hilus, checking for any adhesions between the capsule and the kidney, and for any lesions visible on the surface, for example, nodules, fibrosis, depressions, or infarcts.

Finally, open the stomach along the greater curvature, noting the contents. Remove the contents and examine the internal surface. Open along the small intestines using scissors to the large colon and rectum; note the contents and examine the internal and serosal surfaces and the mesenteric lymph nodes.

Joints

Carefully open the hip, stifle, shoulder and elbow joints, and others if indicated, and examine for abnormal synovial fluid, ruptured, stretched or frayed ligaments, erosion and ulceration of articular cartilage, thickened joint capsules, osteophyte formation and proliferative or thickened synovium. Collect a sample of bone marrow, for example from the mid-shaft of the femur.

Nervous system

Start by removing the head from the body at the atlanto-occipital joint. Make a dorsal midline incision from nose to the foramen magnum and reflect the skin ventrally. Remove the temporal muscles from the skull to expose the bones of the skull (Figure 2.8).

Make cuts through the skull, either with an oscillating saw or a hacksaw (make sure the head is securely held for this, for example in a vice or wrapped in a towel); first cut transversely at the anterior limit of the cranial cavity, slightly posterior to the zygomatic arch. Connect the end of this cut to the foramen magnum. Repeat on the opposite side (Figure 2.9).

Very carefully prise away the calvarium, examining the internal surface. For feline cases, you can instead use bone-cutters to nibble away the skull, starting at the foramen magnum and working forwards to expose the brain (Figures 2.10 and 2.11).

Cut through and reflect the meninges. Working from back to front, gently elevate the brain (or even better, turn the skull upside down and use gravity to help you!) and section each of the cranial nerves

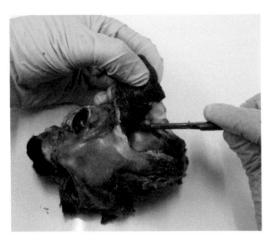

Figure 2.8 Make a dorsal midline incision from nose to the foramen magnum and reflect the skin ventrally. Remove the temporal muscles from the skull to expose the bones of the skull.

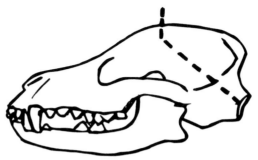

Figure 2.9 To expose the brain, make cuts through the skull, either with an oscillating saw or a hacksaw; first cut transversely at the anterior limit of the cranial cavity, slightly posterior to the zygomatic arch. Connect the end of this cut to the foramen magnum on both sides of the skull.

and the pituitary stalk to free the brain. Transect the olfactory lobes as far cranial as possible. Fix the brain whole in formalin. Free the pituitary gland and collect. If indicated, section the head longitudinally to allow full examination of the nasal cavity and frontal sinuses. Submit the brain fixed and whole for histopathological assessment but be careful it does not become squashed in transport as this distorts the gross architecture. A whole brain, similar to a whole heart, is often the preferred sample as the pathologist can then undertake a thorough assessment of the gross specimen before trimming.

Eyes
To remove the eyes, close the eyelids and use a scalpel to incise through the eyelids around the orbit. With curved scissors, dissect the eyes from the orbits by cutting the extraocular muscles, connective tissue attachments and optic nerve. Collect lacrimal gland tissue if indicated and check for any retrobulbar lesions. Fix whole without incising (formalin is acceptable) and do not attempt to inject formalin into the globe.

If you only occasionally undertake post-mortem examinations, it might be advisable to have a checklist of organs and systems to assess and of samples to take. Table 2.1 provides an example checklist you could have in the practice for such occasions and Table 2.2 a checklist of samples to take for further testing.

Sample collection
The precise samples collected for further testing will vary from case to case and will be dependent to some extent on the clinical history and gross findings. Ideally, tissue samples should be collected from all organs and fixed in 10% neutral buffered formalin – those not submitted in the first instance for histopathology can always be stored in case they are required later. A minimal set of samples for histopathology is indicated in Table 2.2, together with samples which can be taken and stored at $-20\,^{\circ}$C in cases

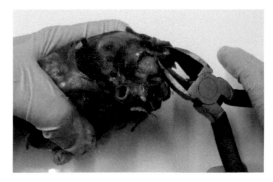

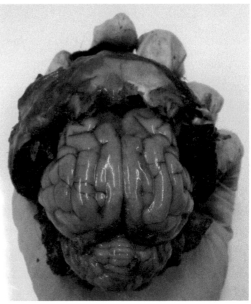

Figure 2.10 and 2.11 **Remove the calvarium to expose the brain.**

where toxicological or polymerase chain reaction (PCR) testing may be indicated (but not viral isolation). Samples for microbial culture can be stored (fresh not fixed) at 4°C. Consider also taking impression smears of lesions for cytology, urine samples and wet preparations of faeces for microscopy – such tests can be valuable for rapid diagnosis.

To achieve the best possible results from histopathology, remember to avoid delayed fixation of samples (samples such as the gastrointestinal [GI] tract, pancreas, kidney and brain in particular) and to use a 10 : 1 volume ratio of formalin : tissue. Remove body fluids, gut contents and so on prior to fixing but do not scrape the tissue surfaces – gentle washing in water is preferable. Take samples no more than 1 cm in thickness, as formalin penetration occurs at approximately 1 mm per hour and central areas of large or thicker samples will not fix quickly enough to preserve tissue detail. If focal lesions are present, take sections from both affected and adjacent normal tissue. Handle the tissues as gently as possible and do not squeeze or crush them with forceps and always remember to label all your sample pots! Finally, when posting samples please remember the packaging must comply with the postal regulations for pathological materials.

Table 2.1 Necropsy checklist

NECROPSY FORM	
Animal details	
Species:	Animal ID:
Breed:	Breeding status:
Sex:	Weight:
Age:	Euthanized?
Date of death:	Date of PME:

Clinical history:	Including previous diagnoses, treatments, group health

PM findings			
Body condition:			
External	✓	Comments	Kidneys, ureter
Body cavities			Urinary bladder
Musculoskeletal			Urethra
Lymph nodes			Trachea
Heart, vessels			Lungs
Liver			Thymus
Gall bladder			Adrenal glands
Pancreas			Gonads
Spleen			Reproductive
Oral cavity			Brain
Oesophagus			Spinal cord
Stomach			Pituitary gland
Small intestine			Bone marrow
Large intestine			Skin
Mammary glands			Joints
Eyes			Other
Thyroid glands			

Additional gross findings:

Photographs?

Table 2.2 **Samples for various further tests**

Toxicology (fresh, frozen)	Minimal set for histopathology (formalin-fixed)	Cytology*, parasitology	Microbial culture‡ (fresh, refrigerated)	Viral isolation†
Liver	Liver	Direct impression smears of lesions	As indicated, e.g. fluids, tissues, swabs	As indicated e.g. 1 cm³ of: lung, liver, kidney, intestine, brain
Kidney	Heart			
Lung	Lung (more than 1 lobe ideally)			
Fat	Kidney	Faecal samples for parasitology		
Stomach content	Spleen			
Urine	GI plus pancreas			
	Any gross lesions!			

Notes:
* If submitting cytology samples for examination by a clinical pathologist, do not place slides in same packaging as formalin-fixed samples – the formalin fumes will cause severe artefacts.
† If viral isolation is indicated it is best to either submit chilled tissues direct to the laboratory, or to take samples into virus transport medium and submit. PCR testing for specific viruses will be possible using tissue samples frozen at – 20°C.
‡ Mycobacteria and some conventional bacteria will survive freezing, but most will not.
Your histopathologist should also be happy to provide you with additional advice regarding any particular case, so if in doubt contact them prior to starting the examination.

Describing gross lesions

Gross pathology is the study of abnormal tissue changes visible to the unaided eye. The aim is to describe what you can see so that another person can clearly picture it without seeing the lesion themselves. Try to avoid identifying what you cannot see – it is probably always best to describe a lesion rather than give it a specific label/diagnosis which you cannot be certain of without examining it under the microscope.

Description not diagnosis

When describing lesions, think about the location, size, colour, shape, consistency, appearance of the cut surface and severity. Try to be simple, concise, clear and to describe precisely, and remember this:

Minimize words, maximize information

Words, lovely words! Here are just a few words you can use to describe gross lesions.

SHAPE   ovoid/oval, spherical, conical, cylindrical, elliptical, triangular, pyramidal, cuboidal, flattened, nodular, reniform, lobulated, tortuous, discoid, punctate, bulbous, wedge, spindle, filiform, mushroom-shaped, domed, irregular, shapeless (is anything truly shapeless?).

COLOUR   be precise, indicate degree, distribution and quality. Also the nature of the colour itself as well as: dark, brilliant, light, pale, mottled, streaked, or stippled. Some are multicoloured, so include them all (red to black). Avoid redundant phrases like 'red in colour' when 'red' will do; avoid phrases which do not actually include a colour (as a resident I used to always get called out for describing something as pale – pale is not a colour).

CONSISTENCY/TEXTURE   hard, tough, firm, pitting, friable, soft, gelatinous, mucoid, dry, inspissated, caseous, crepitant, turgid, stringy, adhesive, gritty, granular, pliable, cartilaginous, bony, semi-solid.

SURFACE   smooth, rough, nodular, haired, shiny, dull, pitted, ulcerated, eroded, elevated, raised, depressed, glistening, rugose, undulant, scaly, covered by exudate (describe the exudate too).

TUBULAR STRUCTURES   can be: patent, dilated, obstructed, obliterated, narrowed, diverticulate, branched, communicating, tortuous.

MODIFYING TERMS   provide additional information: haemorrhagic, necrotizing, suppurative (production of pus), caseous (crumbling, cheese-like consistency), ulcerative, proliferative.

LESION DISTRIBUTION

focal	=	single lesion
multifocal	=	more than one lesion, separated by normal tissue
widespread	=	lesions too numerous to count
diffuse	=	entire tissue is involved
segmental	=	usually related to portions of a tubular organ
coalescing	=	individual lesions merging into one another
disseminated	=	numerous small widely distributed foci (for example, embolic)
transmural	=	throughout all layers of a hollow organ

unilateral/bilateral/bilaterally symmetrical

(My students always wanted to describe things as diffusely multifocal – this is not a thing!)

SIZE   measure the weight and dimensions. People love to compare things size-wise to food items/ fruit. Some love to use chocolates or sweets (I've had Maltesers, Minstrals, Skittles). Some pathologists frown on this. Personally, I do not mind too much, as long as people are specific. It is no use describing something as melon-sized, without including the type of melon; there are nearly 40 different types of melon in the world.

Case study 1

This case study involves a 7-year-old, male (neutered) domestic shorthair cat, previously diagnosed and treated for diabetes mellitus, but who subsequently presented in heart failure (read more about this case by referring to Dobromylskyj and Little, 2021). It illustrates the benefits of correlating clinical and imaging findings, in this case including echocardiography, with gross findings at post-mortem and the subsequent histological assessment.

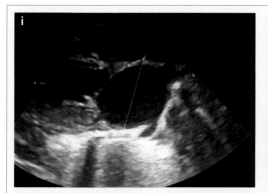
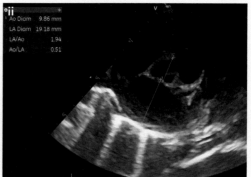

Figure 2.12a Appearance on echocardiography. (i) The right parasternal long axis B-mode ultrasound image of the left heart showing measurement of the dilated left atrium, designated LA max (25 mm). (ii) A right parasternal short-axis B-mode image of the heart base showing measurement of the aortic root and left atrium performed towards the end of diastole. Echocardiography revealed bi-atrial and bi-ventricular dilation with poor myocardial function, and a left atrial to aortic ratio of 1.95:1. There was caudal vena cava dilation, hepatomegaly and ascites.

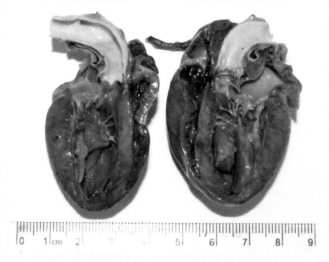

Figure 2.12b Although the heart failure was treated for 5 weeks, the cat then represented recumbent and moribund and was euthanized. Gross assessment of the heart allowed measurements of the ventricular free walls and interventricular septum; right ventricular free wall (RVFW), interventricular septum (IVS) and left ventricular free wall (LVFW) were 2 mm, 4 mm and 8 mm, respectively, giving a ratio of 1 : 2 : 4 (normal ratio is typically considered to be 1 : 3 : 3). It also confirmed dilation of all four chambers and an increased heart weight (27.7 g; approximately 20–21 g is typically considered the upper limit of the normal range for heart weight in cats). This allowed correlation between the findings on echocardiography ante-mortem, and the findings post-mortem, and that this cat demonstrated a dilated phenotype.

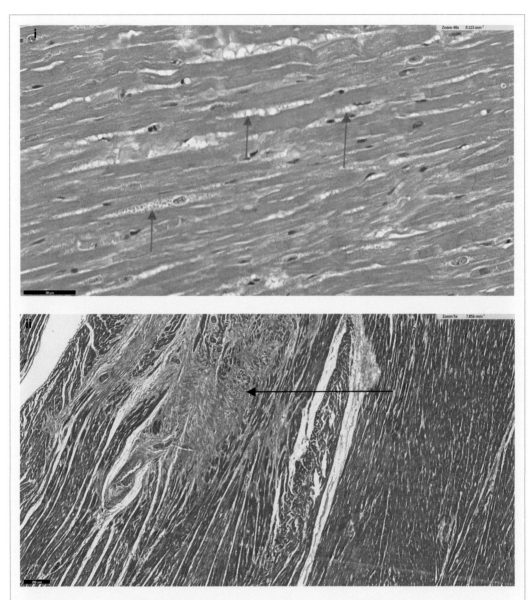

Figure 2.12c Sections through the heart were assessed, stained with (i) HE or (ii) Masson's trichrome for connective tissues. The Masson's trichrome stain showed areas of fibrosis, which would help to explain the poor contractility seen on echocardiography and the abnormalities in cardiac function.

Case study 2

This case study involves an approximately 10-year-old, male crossbreed dog. This case again illustrates the benefits of correlating clinical and imaging findings with gross findings at post-mortem and the microscopic appearance. The clinical history included seizures over the previous five months which had progressed to changes in behaviour, progressive weakness and obtundation.

Neurological examination revealed tetraparesis which was worse on the right side. He circled to the left, and had right-sided proprioceptive deficits, but normal responses on the left. Cranial nerve examination was abnormal with absent menace on the right and absent nasocutaneous response. At this stage, the lesion was neurolocalized to the left forebrain, with neoplastic, infectious and inflammatory causes as potential differential diagnoses.

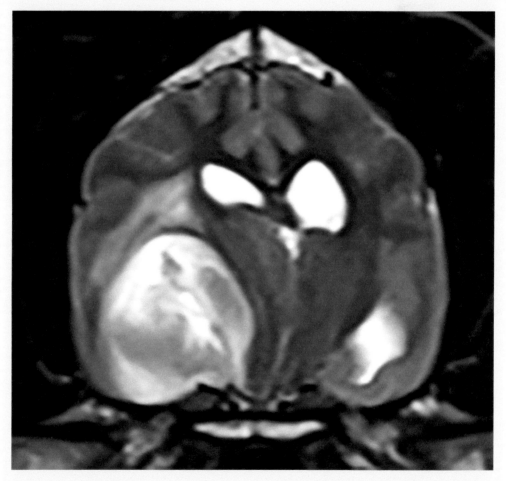

Figure 2.13a MRI of the brain showed a 2 cm × 2 cm mass within the left piriform lobe, causing compression of the lateral ventricle and marked mass effect. At this stage, the most likely differential diagnosis was a neoplasm, most likely a high-grade glioma. Given the poor long-term prognosis, euthanasia was opted for.

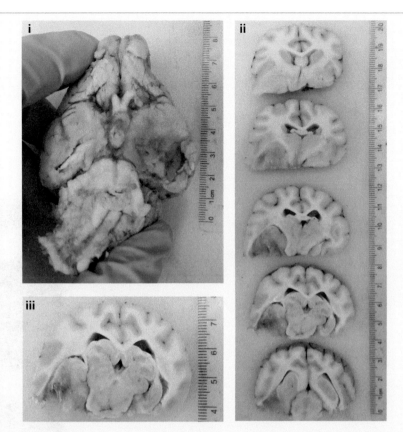

Figure 2.13b Visible from the ventral aspect (i), there is a mass within the left piriform lobe, which on serial sectioning (ii) also contains central cavitated areas, and is reasonably well-demarcated, soft to somewhat gelatinous and mid to dark grey in colour (iii). The mass is compressing and displacing the adjacent brain parenchyma, including shifting to the right and apparent asymmetry.

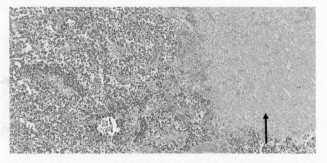

Figure 2.13c Microscopic examination of sections from the brain at the level of the left piriform lobe confirms a glioma, with histological features consistent with an oligodendroglioma. Increased mitotic activity, necrosis (black arrow) and microvascular proliferation as well as the degree of anisokaryosis were suggestive of a high-grade neoplasm in this case, as was suspected from the MRI appearance (graded according to Koehler et al., 2018).

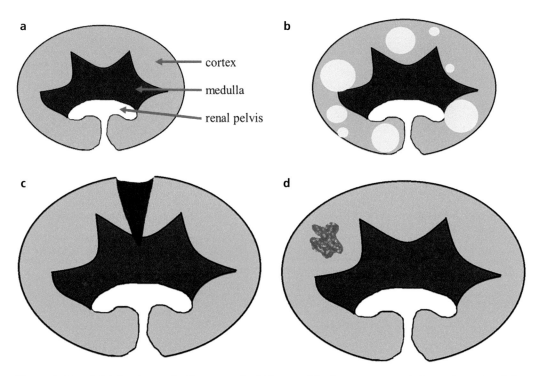

Figure 2.14a–d (a) A schematic diagram of a kidney, with the cortex, medulla and renal pelvis labelled. (b–d) Images of different lesions arising in the kidney.

Self-assessment: gross lesion descriptions

Have a try at a gross description for each lesion shown in Figure 2.14. Remember to think about the number, shape, colour, demarcation and the lesion distribution.

The answers are available on page 170.

Self-assessment: quick quiz questions

1. What are the main organs and structures which make up the 'pluck'?
2. What does it mean if a portion of lung tissue floats in formalin?
3. How would you check for the presence of negative pressure in the thoracic cavity?
4. What is the normal ratio of thickness of the right ventricular free wall (RVFW), interventricular septum and left ventricular free wall (LVFW)?
5. How would you check for patency of the bile duct?

The answers are available on page 171.

Biopsy types with regards to tumour grading and margin assessment

3

Introduction

There are several different types of biopsy and it is really important that clinicians recognize the pros and cons of each type when deciding which to perform in any given situation. This includes what, if any, limitations the chosen biopsy type might place on the pathologist and what they may or may not be able to tell you based on the sample submitted. We look at lymph nodes as a good example, and some tumours including those arising in mammary tissues and bone. In the second section, we look at margin assessment, different types and what they can and cannot tell you, as well as factors which impact on their assessment.

Different types of biopsies, and their pros and cons

An excisional biopsy, for example, of a mass-lesion, will entail submission of the entire mass, and will enable assessment of the margins as well as a diagnosis and an accurate tumour grade, where appropriate. Even excisional biopsies can vary in their nature, from those with very narrow margins, where the mass is essentially 'shelled out', to those removed with wider margins with curative intent, to more radical samples like limb amputations.

There are also various forms of incisional biopsies, which is where only part of a mass or lesion, or a representative tissue sample from an organ such as the liver, is submitted for microscopic assessment. Incisional biopsies can range from wedge samples through to smaller punch and Tru-cut needle biopsies.

For some sites such as the gastrointestinal tract, samples might be full-thickness surgical biopsies or endoscopic biopsies predominantly composed of the mucosa. Suction biopsies obtained via a catheter from the urinary bladder will probably yield mostly mucosa and therefore probably less information than a full-thickness sample of the bladder wall taken at surgery.

These various forms of biopsy samples each have their own benefits and potential drawbacks, both clinically but also from the pathologist's point of view. This is not to say the type of biopsy a clinician chooses to perform should be determined solely by the pathologist! But it is important to bear in mind that some types of biopsies have their limitations, which should be considered when planning a sampling technique.

Liver biopsies (wedge versus Tru-cut) and gastrointestinal biopsies (surgical versus endoscopic) will be covered in more detail in Chapter 4. Here we will look at some other examples where limitations of incisional versus excisional biopsies can be nicely seen.

Lymph nodes

Lymph nodes make a really good example. They may be biopsied because they are enlarged, or as part of staging of a neoplastic disease; as such the potential questions being asked of the pathologist are typically 'Is this a reactive lymph node or is it lymphoma?' or 'Is there evidence of metastatic disease X?' Traditionally biopsies from lymph nodes can be either of the entire node (excisional) or part of the node (incisional, for example, wedge or needle biopsy). A brief review of the histology of a normal or reactive lymph node is shown in Figure 3.1; a normal or reactive lymph node will have an intact capsule, a subcapsular sinus (although in a reactive lymph node this may well be compressed), and a distinct cortex and medulla; a reactive lymph node will also have prominent lymphoid follicle formation, potentially with visible germinal centres.

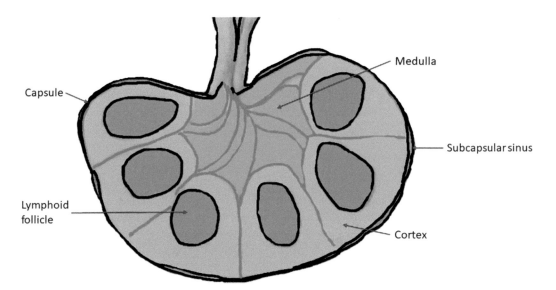

Figure 3.1 Schematic representation of a reactive lymph node, with capsule, subcapsular sinus, medulla and cortex containing prominent lymphoid follicles.

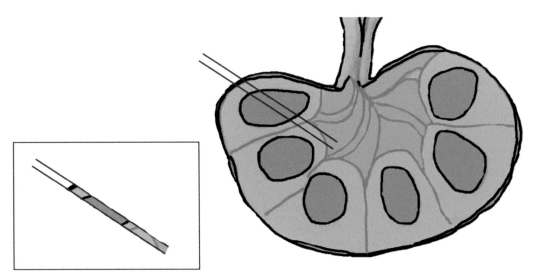

Figure 3.2 Schematic representation of a reactive lymph node undergoing needle biopsy; the inset demonstrates what parts of the lymph node would be present within the needle biopsy for assessment by the pathologist, compared to the entire node (present in an excisional biopsy).

Figure 3.2 shows this reactive lymph node undergoing a needle biopsy, and the inset demonstrates what parts of the lymph node would be present within that needle biopsy core for assessment by the pathologist, compared to the entire node which would be present in an excisional biopsy. In this case, the core contains areas of the capsule, compressed subcapsular sinus, a lymphoid follicle and part of the surrounding cortex as well as a small area of medulla, which would suggest to the pathologist that the lymph node architecture was retained, assuming this sample was fully representative of the whole node.

In some forms of lymphoma, the pathological changes present within the lymph node are diffuse and completely efface the normal lymph node architecture, for example as seen in a diffuse large B-cell lymphoma (DLBCL – see Figure 3.3), therefore a needle/incisional biopsy would most likely result in an accurate diagnosis.

However, some forms of lymphoma are not diffuse, but rather nodular in their histological appearance, and the diagnosis of these forms of lymphoma relies heavily on seeing these changes to the normal lymph node architecture (see Figure 3.4). In these cases, there is potential for a needle biopsy to be misleading, and even an incisional biopsy may not allow for a confident diagnosis (for incisional biopsies, the process of sampling itself often appears to disrupt the normal lymph node architecture, making it difficult for the pathologist to assess).

Metastatic disease is also often focal in nature, therefore submitting the entire lymph node is more likely to detect its presence than a needle or incisional biopsy, as more of the node is histologically assessed (Figure 3.5 – red oval is the metastatic lesion).

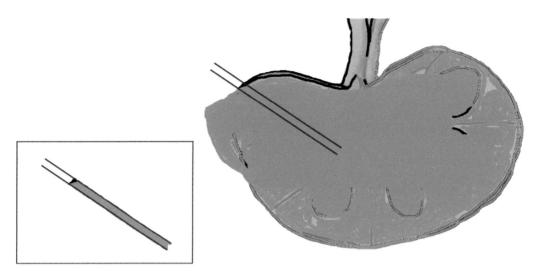

Figure 3.3 Schematic representation of a lymph node effaced by a diffuse pathological process such as a diffuse large B-cell lymphoma, undergoing needle biopsy; the inset demonstrates what parts of the lymph node would be present within the needle biopsy for assessment.

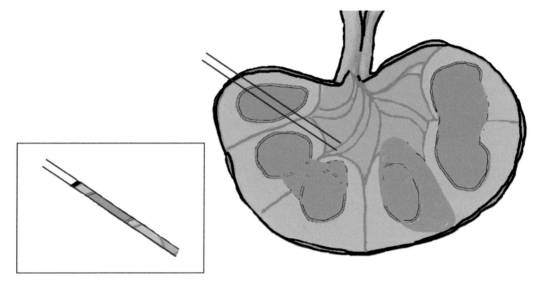

Figure 3.4 Schematic representation of a lymph node with a nodular form of lymphoma (such as a follicular lymphoma), undergoing needle biopsy; the inset demonstrates what parts of the lymph node would be present within the needle biopsy for assessment.

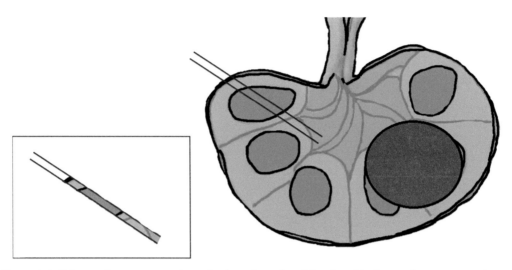

Figure 3.5 Schematic representation of a lymph node with a focal lesion such as metastatic disease (red oval), undergoing needle biopsy; in this case the needle biopsy has not sampled the part of the node containing the metastatic lesion.

Challenges with tumours and incisional biopsy types

Bone lesions

Many bone lesions will be sampled via needle biopsies to obtain a diagnosis prior to potentially radical surgery. The biopsy is often guided by radiographic changes and with concern for any pathological fractures arising. It is important to remember that alongside the potentially neoplastic process, there will also be often widespread concurrent reactive and/or secondary changes present including necrosis and osteolysis of pre-existing bone, reactive fibroplasia and inflammation, as well as sometimes marked periosteal new bone formation as the bone attempts to counteract the instability caused by the presence of the tumour and bone loss. Samples, if fully representative, will therefore often be composed of a mixture of these tissues, including necrotic bone, new reactive bone and bone or osteoid matrix potentially associated with a tumour. Because the reactive and secondary changes are often florid and more superficial, it is not uncommon for needle biopsies to not contain any direct evidence of the neoplastic lesion itself, but this does not mean neoplasia can be excluded from the differential list (Figure 3.6).

Mammary tumours

Incisional biopsies of mammary tumours, be that Tru-cut, punch biopsy or wedge, can also be misleading. Mammary tumours undergoing early malignant transformation often only have focal areas of peripherally infiltrative growth, while the remainder of the mass appears histologically fairly benign – such foci may be missed by incisional biopsies, leading to an underestimation of a tumour's malignancy. Incisional biopsies will also contain less (or none) of the surrounding tissues, lessening the opportunity to detect any lymphatic or blood vessel invasion indicative of potential metastatic spread. The classification of mammary tumours depends in part on the different cell/tissues present, and these may also not be fully represented in incisional biopsies.

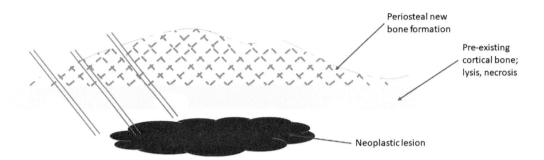

Figure 3.6 Schematic representation of a bone neoplasm, with the area of neoplasia in red. The overlying pre-existing cortical bone is lytic, and there is a large area of periosteal new bone formation. Needle biopsies represented by parallel blue lines, illustrating how the underlying neoplastic lesion may be missed during sampling, or only present in relatively small parts of the sampled tissues, alongside necrotic/lytic bone and reactive new bone formation.

Tumour grading

Incisional biopsies can also be potentially misleading in terms of tumour grading. Some tumour grading schemes include features such as the mitotic count, and/or the presence and extent of any necrosis, and such features can vary between different parts of a tumour. For example, an incisional biopsy may not include any areas of necrosis in a soft tissue sarcoma (Figure 3.7), and when a follow-up excisional biopsy is submitted for assessment, necrosis is seen to be present resulting in a higher histological grade. For mast cell tumours, mitotic counts can vary between different parts of the mass, and localization of a tumour within the dermis, subcutis or both can affect the grade/prognosis – absence of any surround-

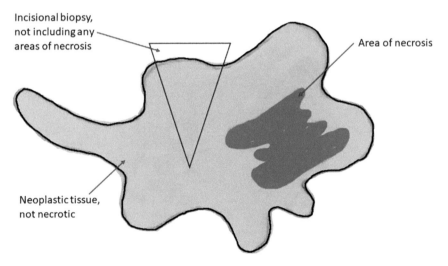

Figure 3.7 Schematic representation of a tumour such as a soft tissue sarcoma, with an area of necrosis in dark grey. An incisional (wedge) biopsy is represented by blue lines, illustrating how the area of necrosis may be missed, resulting in a lower histological grade than would be suggested by an excisional biopsy.

ing tissues within an incisional biopsy sample can make it difficult or impossible to assess the precise location of the mass.

Different forms of biopsy samples have benefits and also potential drawbacks, both clinically and also diagnostically, and this will vary depending on the site or lesion and the questions being asked. A better understanding of the potential limitations of different forms of biopsy will hopefully allow for the most appropriate type to be chosen for any individual case, and also help in interpreting the subsequent histopathological report. If in any doubt, you can always discuss the case with a pathologist prior to performing the biopsy sampling.

Margin assessment

This is a big and important topic, but to begin with there are some key concepts to get across. It is simply not possible to microscopically assess the whole volume of a tumour; see the case study for an example of why this is not practical.

Case study

If we use an example of a mass which is 5 cm in diameter, the volume of tumour would be 65.45 cm^3. The whole surface of a tumour, that is, the 'margins' for our 5 cm diameter mass would be 78.54 cm^2. If we say a single block could hold a slice of tissue 2.5 cm $\times$ 3 cm $\times$ 0.3 cm, then the maximum area of tumour which can theoretically be contained within a cassette is 7.5 cm^2.

For our 5 cm diameter mass, 0.3 cm interval 'slices' would result in 16.66 slices through the mass. At its widest point, a 'slice' would need six blocks to contain all of the tissue. It would require 54 blocks to trim in all of the tissue. And of course, if each block contains tissue 0.3 cm thick, and each section on a slide is only 4 μm thick, that equates to 750 sections per block, making 40,500 slides to look at all of that 5 cm diameter tumour, and that does not include any of the surrounding tissues.

Taking this example a little further, if we say each slide can take 1 minute to scan digitally, that would take 675 hours, or just over 28 days to scan that one case, and this is before a pathologist has even looked at a single slide. Each slide can take 1–4 gigabytes of storage space, meaning we would require a minimum of 40.5 terabytes to store the images for this 5 cm diameter mass!

What we do is therefore inevitably a compromise between the impossible (as illustrated by the case study above) and the practical, in terms of financial costs, numbers of slides, time to assess and the accuracy of the assessment, while deriving the most useful information for the veterinary surgeon, the owner and their animal. Another issue is that the terminology used is often very muddled; we clearly need to work towards a common understanding and a more universal vocabulary, and this can only come from working together. As always, communication is key and needs to flow freely in all directions; between oncologist, surgeon, possibly an imager and a nurse packing any sample, and the pathologist and their technical teams.

Margins, put most simply, are what helps to determine whether there is local disease control or the likelihood of local recurrence. However, **it is an imprecise process**, as you will see. From the surgeon, it helps to know what the surgical approach or intent was – was the sample taken for initial diagnosis only, for the purposes of de-bulking the disease, to reduce the process to microscopic disease only, or is it an attempt at curative excision? It can help for the surgeon to describe briefly the technique used, that is, was this an incisional / intra-capsular biopsy, or an excisional sample? If excisional, is it intended to be marginal, wide, or radical, and have any margins been submitted for assessment? It also really helps to know whether there were tumour free margins grossly as assessed by the surgeon. This is of course rather different to histological tumour free margins (HTFM).

Surgeons can also greatly aid pathologists by indicating any areas of particular concern, and by identifying those and the margins, for example by the use of surgical inks or suture tags. Fixation alters the gross appearance of tissues, and also distorts tissues in relation to one another, meaning that something which looked obvious at the time of surgery, may no longer be so obvious once it reaches the laboratory, and so clear indication of these areas is critical. The surgeon is clearly in the best position to identify areas of concern and also the orientation of the tissue sample once removed from the patient.

Practical tips on the use of suture tags
A few notes on the use of suture tags.

1. Please do not tie them or bed them in overly tight – we have to remove any suture tags before embedding and sectioning, as otherwise when the suture material comes into contact with the microtome blade, it catches and simply tears the tissues and wrecks the section.
2. Please note the colour and/or number of tags (single tag, double tag, long ends, short ends and so on) as a means to differentiate between multiple tags on a sample, but do not identify them by solely their material type. Laboratory personnel are not familiar with the likes of Prolene or Vicryl, and so this does not allow for them to confidently distinguish between types of tags on an individual sample and to correlate them with the clinical notes.

Pathologists can also help and should take note that a margin is more than just a number (a somewhat arbitrary number at that, which we will look at next). When reporting margins, pathologists should ideally incorporate the distance between neoplastic tissue and the margin (histological tumour free margin [HTFM]), the degree of invasiveness of the tumour, and the types of tissues and location of any fascial planes that make up this margin. Pathologists can also help by avoiding the use of vague and undefined terms such as 'close' or 'narrow', 'clean' or 'dirty'. These are at best arbitrary, and are poorly if at all defined, and there is currently a general lack of data to support any particular given values.

Each tumour and tumour type is unique and each will have their own growth habits and natural history within a given patient. We make an assumption that they will all behave in a certain way, because without these assumptions we would never be able to formulate any treatment plans or discuss prognoses in a meaningful way, but it is important to remember they are only that – assumptions! Each patient and each tumour are unique and even within each tumour there will be different populations of tumour cells behaving in different ways – slightly mind boggling when you stop and think about it.

Inking

Inking is one means of identification – and this might be to allow for orientation of a sample, to identify all margins, or to identify certain areas of concern. Inking helps the pathologist be more confident that the margin observed histologically *is* the margin of surgically excised tissues. It is best done by the surgeon at the time of surgery and on fresh tissues. The surgeon knows best the areas of most concern and the tissue/sample orientation in relation to the arrangement *in vivo*. Inking fresh tissue also avoids some of the issues of tissue contraction.

There is growing recognition of the importance of inking, yet there is limited practical information about the technique. Below are hopefully some easy-to-follow steps on how to apply the ink before submitting the sample to the laboratory.

In terms of equipment, very little is actually required, but it is important to use suitable ink, such as the Davidson Marking System Tissue Marking Dyes. Please make sure the correct ink is used; using the wrong type of ink may potentially damage laboratory equipment, as well as not being visible in the histological sections. In addition to ink, all that is needed is space (and time), gloves, swabs and cotton buds.

Not all the different coloured inks are equally good. If the mass or lesion is pigmented, for example a melanoma (and oral and digits in particular), then avoid black ink and other dark colours. Try to avoid pale colours (for example, yellow) which do not show well in the histological sections, or pink and purple as these do not always contrast well with HE staining. As a general rule, green and blue tend to be the colours that show most clearly in the histological sections. And importantly, if using multiple colours, ensure you choose colours which are clearly different to one another, and indicate on the submission form what each colour indicates. Figures 3.8 to 3.10 show a step by step process of applying of ink to a surgical specimen. This might be all of the deep and lateral margins, or a particular area the surgeon is concerned about and wishes to highlight to the pathologist. Remember to indicate what/where you have inked on the submission form. Figure 3.11 shows how it should appear in the histological sections when correctly applied.

There are also some things to avoid, and these include not incising into neoplastic tissues prior to ink application and avoiding incising into margins once inked – these both allow the ink to penetrate into areas of the tissues other than the margin – this is a real problem and a technical limitation of inking. The dissection of ink along fascial planes or inadvertently adhering to other surfaces is a fairly common issue and one which can impact on margin assessment. As well as ink being where it should not be (Figure 3.12), sometimes poor application of ink means that ink is absent from where it should be, and this is also a limitation of the technique.

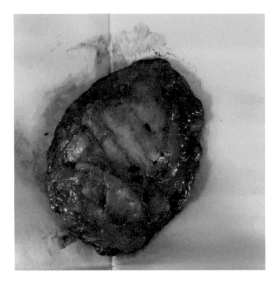

Figure 3.8 Blot the sample so that the surface you want to ink is dry, using gauze swabs.

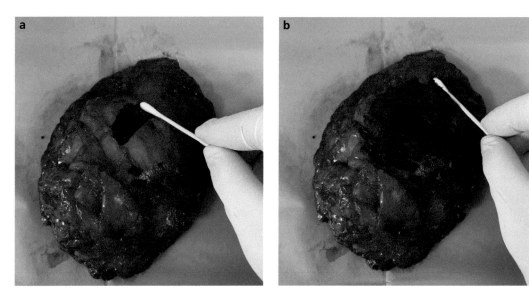

Figure 3.9 Apply drops of the ink onto a cotton bud. Using a rolling motion, use the cotton bud to paint the margins (that is, the cut surfaces you wish to be histologically assessed). A wooden applicator stick can also be used. Do not pour the dye on to the surface, just apply as if 'painting'.

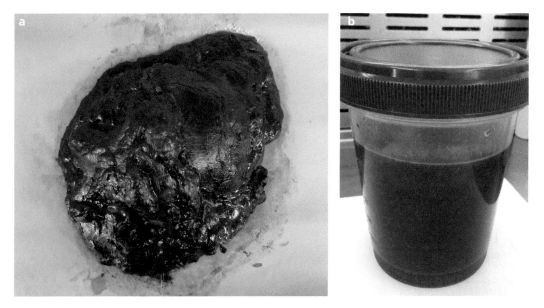

Figure 3.10 Once inking is complete, leave the sample to dry for 15–20 minutes before placing into formalin as per normal. Do not worry, some of the ink will come off and colour the formalin.

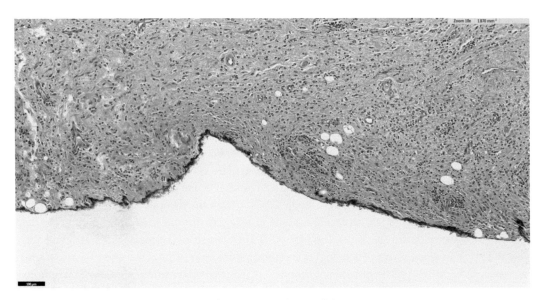

Figure 3.11 Ink where it should be. Clear green inking of deep margin.

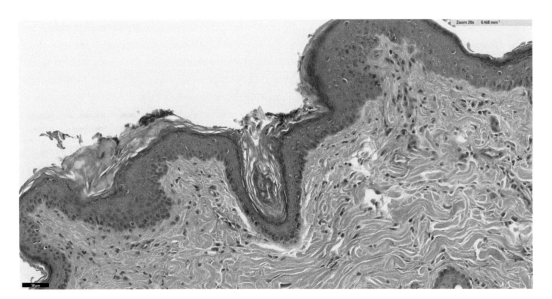

Figure 3.12 Ink where it probably should not be: keratin layer overlying the epidermis, it seems to get everywhere.

Artefacts

There are changes occurring within tissues that mean that the absolute margin as it appears in real life does not directly equate to the margin seen grossly post-excision/pre-fixation, or post-fixation, and most definitely does not equate to the distance measured on the slide. This means that the number supplied to you by the pathologist is only a guide, and not an absolute value in itself.

Tissue shrinkage in particular happens at different stages in the process:

- post-surgical contraction
- during fixation
- during processing
- during trimming.

To complicate things further, different tissues shrink at different rates within the same sample, meaning that the changes are not proportional to one another. This can also alter the overall shape of the sample and distort the relationships between different tissue types and planes. It may also vary between species and between different parts of the body, depending on the tissues present. In the immediate post-excision/pre-fixation period, for example, tissue shrinkage occurs due to myofibril contractility and tissue elasticity when those tissues are released from surrounding structures, and skin, muscle and fascia may all 'shrink' at different rates. Pathologists are not doubting your surgical margins of excision when we report such small-sounding distances, I promise – if you say you removed with 2 cm margins, we believe you! Even if on our slide they measure much, much less; remember that the number we supply you with is a guide only.

Other artefacts with the potential to impact on margin assessment include incomplete fixation as that means some parts of the tissues change shape more than others. The use of too small a sample pot causes three-dimensional distortion of the sample (as discussed in Chapter 1), obscuring the true shape of the sample and the relationship between a mass and any margins submitted. During trimming and sectioning there is also the risk of dissociation between tissue types/planes, compounded by differential rates of tissue shrinkage. Placement of tissues in cassettes can also inadvertently cause distortion of tissues if too large a section is placed in one cassette. Processing further causes shrinkage and distortion of differing degrees between tissue types. Sectioning can induce further artefacts, such as tissue folding, splitting or contraction and dissociation of tissues; if severe enough, sections have to be re-cut.

Different types of margins

There are different techniques for the assessment of margins. It is important that you understand what they each entail, and their limitations/advantages.

Cross-sectional or radial

Cross-sectional or radial is probably the most common form of margin assessment. It involves assessing a full cross-section through the sample at the widest point, typically together with two additional quarter sections taken perpendicular to the cross-section. This enables assessment of four 'lateral' margins and one 'deep' margin (Figures 3.13 and 3.14). This can be modified as a technique for larger masses, where a full cross-section is sub-divided into smaller areas to fit a tissue cassette.

The cross-sectional technique is cost effective, easy and, importantly, allows for measurement of the margins. However, its disadvantages include an assumption of symmetrical and expansile growth of all masses in a centrifugal fashion from the centre. It also inevitably only evaluates a portion of the marginal tissues, meaning that 'fingers' of tumour tissue will potentially be missed. Figure 3.15 illustrates one such mass viewed from above, which when trimmed one way appears to have complete lateral margins but when trimmed another way appears incompletely excised, with neoplastic cells extending

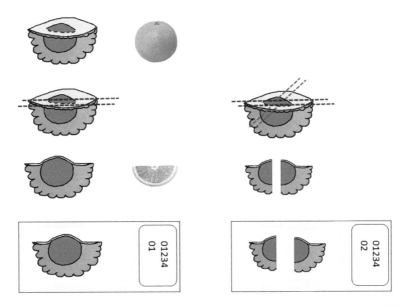

Figure 3.13 Schematic diagram showing cross-sectional technique from mass to slides.

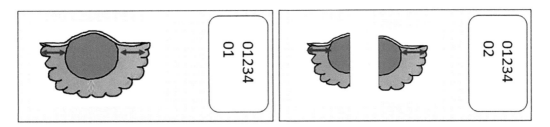

Figure 3.14 Margin measurement for cross-sectional technique; the one green arrow is the deep margin and the four purple arrows are the four 'lateral' margins.

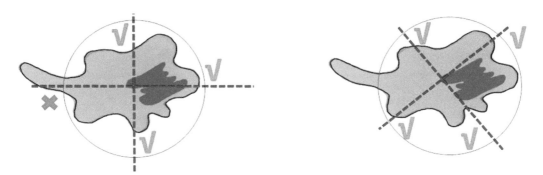

Figure 3.15 Cross-sectional technique has the potential to miss incomplete margins of excision, depending on where the sections are trimmed from.

to one of the lateral margins. Detection of the incomplete margin depends on where the cross-sections are taken from.

Bread loaf or pie

Bread loaf or pie is in some ways similar to cross-sectional, but rather than four, there are multiple slices taken, either in the form of slicing a loaf of bread or dividing a pie. This technique means more of the marginal tissues are assessed, and the pathologist can adapt this to focus on any areas of concern flagged at submission. The more slices examined, in theory the better the assessment, however, the approach is limited by the cost of trimming, processing, sectioning and staining larger numbers of sections, and by the cost of the pathologist's time in assessing them all.

Tangential/shaved/orange peel

Tangential/shaved/orange peel is less commonly used, and the variety of names also causes some confusion. The premise is that the technicians or pathologists 'shave off' only the marginal tissues, like peeling the skin off an orange, and these are what are assessed microscopically by the pathologist. The obvious advantage is that there is theoretically complete assessment of all marginal tissues (Figure 3.16). The important thing to note is that pathologists cannot **measure** margins when they are trimmed in this way. The result becomes binary, black or white, either tumour is present in the marginal tissues, or it is not. Please do not request the pathologist then measures margins trimmed in this way, as it is not possible!

Tumour bed

The tumour bed technique in some ways is a bit similar to tangential margins, although the tissue is obtained by the surgeon from the tumour bed and submitted separately from the main mass or sample. It does not assess the whole margin but allows the surgeon to focus on areas of most concern. This also gives a binary result, with samples being either positive or negative for the presence of neoplastic tissues, and so these also cannot be measured. One other potential limitation of such techniques is when it becomes difficult to distinguish between an individual or small number of neoplastic cells from normal or reactive ones – for example mast cells at the edge of a mast cell tumour, or fibroblast-like cells at the

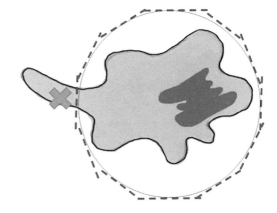

Figure 3.16 The same mass as in Figure 3.15, this time trimmed to produce tangential margins, this technique would detect the incomplete margin, however, it also involves three times as many slides. Note that these illustrations are only 2D, whereas in real life tumours are 3D – thus rather than the circumference it is the surface area which is being trimmed and assessed.

edge of a sarcoma. This is because the tissue architecture and information gained from the growth pattern of the tumour are mostly absent in such thin samples of tissue, so those visual clues are no longer available to the pathologist.

Of course, we are making a number of assumptions here once again. One of those is Halsted's oncologic concept of systematic 'centrifugal' tumour growth, and another is that the surgeon must remove all of the tumour in order to cure the patient. There are, of course, examples of tumours which do not recur despite apparently incomplete margins and also vice versa, which may in part come back to the quandary of differentiating between normal and neoplastic cells, and also the process of 'remission'.

More recently, there has been a move to suggest a different approach, based on the Union for International Cancer Control guidelines. Simplified, this is:

R0 = resection with surgical margins both macroscopically and microscopically negative for neoplastic cells
R1 = surgical margin with microscopic evidence of neoplastic cells but macroscopically normal*
R2 = macroscopically residual tumour
*incomplete histologic excision, satellite tumour cell populations distant to tumour, lymphatic or venous or perineural invasion, lymph node or microscopic distant metastasis
OR
R0 = HTFM ≥ 1 mm; R1 = HTFM < 1 mm; R2 = intralesional tumoral resection

Another group is the Veterinary Cancer Guidelines and Protocols (VCGP). The goal of the VCGP is the standardization of tumour evaluation and reporting, as there are currently no published guidelines for veterinary pathologists to follow. The 'VCGP creates these guidelines and protocols acting as centralized resources for veterinary anatomic and clinical pathologists to assist in reporting and also in gathering relevant information about aggressive tumours' (www.vcgp.com).

Self-assessment: multiple choice questions

1. In which of the following types of margin assessment can the lateral and deep margins be measured?
   a Tumour bed technique
   b Cross-sectional
   c Tangential
   d Shaved

2. What is the histological tumour free margin?
   a The distance between the mass and the surgical margin as seen grossly at the time of surgery.
   b The distance between the neoplastic tissue and the margin as seen microscopically.
   c The degree of tumour invasiveness.
   d The distance between the mass and the surgical margin as seen grossly by the pathologist once the sample is completely fixed.

3. What is the relationship between the gross margin you see surgically and the distance measured on the slide by the pathologist?
   a They are the same in size.
   b The gross margin is smaller than the distance measured on the slide.
   c The gross margin is larger than the distance measured on the slide by a factor of at least 10.
   d The gross margin is larger than the distance measured on the slide but the factor varies.

4. What type of margin assessment theoretically allows complete assessment of all marginal tissues?
   a Cross-sectional
   b Bread loafing
   c Tangential
   d Pie

5. Using suture tags to indicate areas of interest is a good idea, but you must:
   a make sure you bed them in nice and tight, so they do not fall off in transit
   b make sure they are all the same colour
   c remember to include what type of suture material you have used
   d none of the above.

The answers are available on page 171.

Self-assessment: case study

The patient is a 9-year-old, male (neutered) Golden retriever dog, who has presented with a mass on the distal left forelimb. The client says the mass has suddenly appeared in the last week, is increasing in size quickly and that the dog is self-traumatizing it. On a fine needle aspirate you diagnose the mass as a mast cell tumour. Palpation of the left pre-scapular lymph node reveals it is slightly larger than the right pre-scapular lymph node, so you obtain a further fine needle aspirate from the right pre-scapular lymph node for submission to the laboratory, and plan to perform a surgical excision of the mass. The anatomical location is difficult, as you feel margins will be difficult to achieve.

- When submitting the fine needle aspirate sample from the right pre-scapular lymph node for cytological assessment, how should you package this (think back to Chapter 1)?
- The surgically excised mass is too large for a routine sample pot, what should you do (think back to Chapter 1)?
- You are particularly worried about the deep margins, and one of the lateral margins; what can you do to help the pathologist accurately assess those particular margins?

The answers are available on page 172.

Gastrointestinal and liver biopsies

4

CHAPTER SUMMARY

Gastrointestinal biopsies
> Pros and cons of endoscopic versus surgical biopsies
> Case study 1
> Case study 2
> Submitting GI biopsy samples
> Interpretation of inflammatory lesions – WSAVA
> > guidelines
> What we cannot tell you

Liver biopsies
> Pros and cons of Tru-cut versus surgical biopsies
> How does the pathologist assess a liver biopsy?
> If inflammatory, is this a reactive hepatopathy or a
> > true hepatitis?
> Copper and canine chronic hepatopathy

Self-assessment: multiple choice questions

Introduction

This chapter looks at biopsies from the gastrointestinal (GI) tract and the liver in more detail, particularly in terms of the different types of biopsies and any limitations the form of biopsy may have in terms of the diagnostic information obtainable. We will look at how pathologists interpret inflammatory conditions in the GI tract, and how we approach liver biopsies also. Feline intestinal lymphoma can be a particular diagnostic challenge for both pathologists and clinicians, as can chronic hepatitis in dogs, and so we will take a closer look at both conditions.

Gastrointestinal biopsies

Pros and cons of endoscopic versus surgical biopsies

Biopsies from the GI tract are a good example of an instance when the biopsy type may impact what can be diagnosed, and a good knowledge and understanding of the differences between the types is important when deciding which technique to use for any given case. Biopsies comprised of mucosa only (that is, endoscopic biopsies) may miss some diagnoses where the main or only pathological process involves the deeper layers of the intestinal wall, while other histological features or diseases are more reliably assessed when the deeper layers are also present.

With full-thickness samples there is also simply more tissue for the pathologist to look at (Figure 4.1), including more of the mucosa as well as the submucosa and muscular layers. Figure 4.2 illustrates which areas might be included in endoscopic biopsies taken from the same portion of intestines.

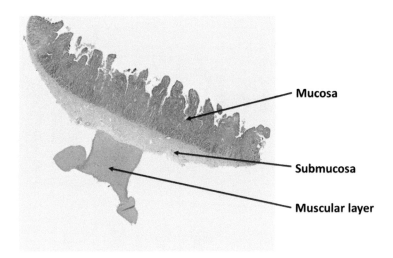

Figure 4.1 Illustration of a full-thickness small intestinal biopsy, with the different layers.

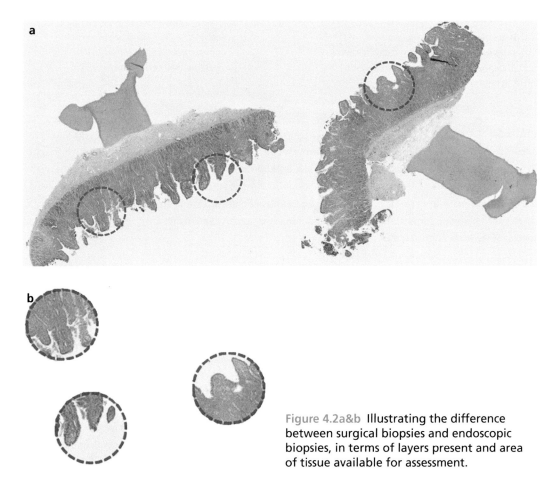

Figure 4.2a&b Illustrating the difference between surgical biopsies and endoscopic biopsies, in terms of layers present and area of tissue available for assessment.

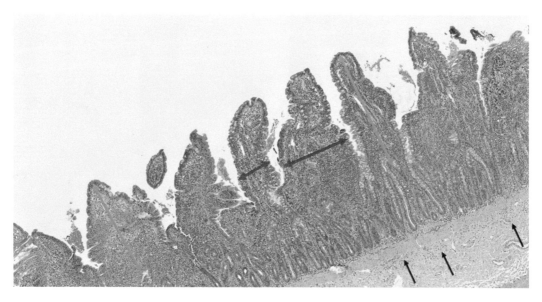

Figure 4.3 This full-thickness sample allows for several adjacent villi to be compared to one another in terms of length (light blue arrows) and width (red), and also compared to the crypts in the deeper lamina propria. It also shows infiltration of the submucosa by small lymphocytes, a feature associated with feline low-grade alimentary lymphoma (small cell, diffuse type – dark blue arrows), which would not be apparent from endoscopic biopsy samples.

Full-thickness samples are normally better orientated, and this allows for a more confident assessment of the architecture of the tissues. For example, assessment of villous morphology requires comparison between villi and crypts, and may be more accurate in well-orientated, full-thickness biopsies (Figure 4.3). While it is still usually feasible in endoscopic biopsies where both villous and deep lamina propria are present, it is not possible at all in more superficial endoscopic biopsies where only villous lamina propria is present, due to the absence of crypts (Figure 4.4).

Limiting the samples to the mucosa (that is, endoscopic) means that a number of diseases may be missed when sampling, either due to the small biopsy size or because they are not located in the mucosal layer. Some relatively common diseases may be more reliably diagnosed by full-thickness samples compared to endoscopic biopsies, because confirmation of the diagnosis may rely on features seen within the deeper intestinal layers as well as in the mucosa (if indeed they are even present in the mucosa), although a suspicion may be raised by the histological appearance of endoscopic biopsies. These conditions include neoplastic and non-neoplastic processes, with some examples and case studies listed below. Full-thickness samples are also needed to identify lesions involving nerve bundles or ganglion cells, as well as other lesions such as smooth muscle hypertrophy.

Lymphangiectasia

A good example of this would be lymphangiectasia, either congenital or acquired, which is one cause of protein-losing enteropathy in the dog. The precise underlying cause often cannot be confirmed, however, it has been suggested that apparently acquired lymphangiectasia may be the result of leakage of lymph (perhaps from a congenitally compromised lymphatic system) and the subsequent

a

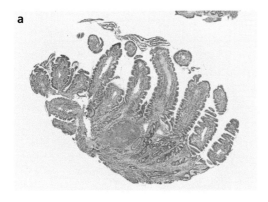

b

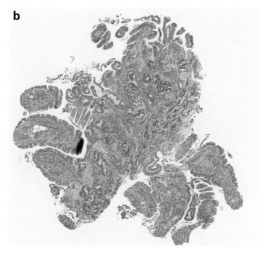

c

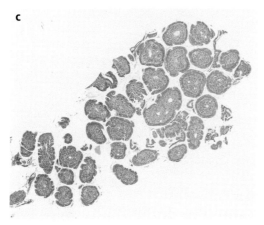

Figure 4.4a–c (a) A good quality endoscopy biopsy sample – there are villi and crypts present for assessment, and orientation is good. (b) An endoscopic biopsy sample of adequate quality. Although there are villi and some crypts present, the orientation is sub-optimal. (c) An endoscopic biopsy sample that is composed of villi only. It is not possible to accurately assess villous morphology from this sample, nor can the deeper lamina propria be assessed.

granulomatous response that causes obstruction, which then in turn further aggravates the lymphatic abnormality. Concurrent inflammatory changes within the mucosa may be surprisingly minimal to mild with this condition, with the only suggestive change being dilation of central lacteals within villi (Figure 4.5a) – but this is a non-specific finding and can also be seen to some extent with other forms of enteropathies. This feature of central lacteal dilation may even be missed if too few samples have been obtained. The more striking and definitive changes are often to be seen within the deeper intestinal layers and/or the associated mesentery (Figure 4.5b), which will only be present in full-thickness biopsy samples.

Feline gastrointestinal eosinophilic sclerosing fibroplasia
Feline gastrointestinal eosinophilic sclerosing fibroplasia is another example where the key histological findings are mostly or entirely to be seen within the deeper intestinal layers – this is significant because this condition often presents as an intestinal mass with mesenteric lymph node involvement, but is not neoplastic in nature. Biopsies from adjacent intestines are reported to be often relatively normal in this condition. To read more about a particular case of this entity see Davidson et al. (2016). In this open access case report, there is correlation between ultrasound images, gross appearance at surgery and the histopathological findings, as well as a good review of the current literature.

Case study 1

A case of suspected acquired lymphangiectasia in a 5-year-old, male (neutered) Staffordshire bull terrier dog. This dog presented with a clinical history of chronic diarrhoea, which was associated with hypoproteinaemia, lymphopaenia, hypocalcaemia, and hypocholesterolaemia.

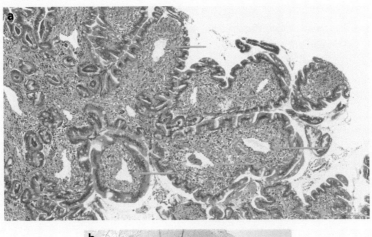

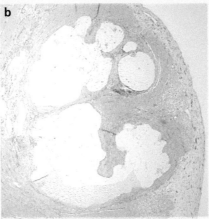

Figure 4.5 (a) In this high-power view of the mucosa, the inflammation within the villous and deep lamina propria was mild, and composed of lymphocytes, plasma cells and smaller numbers of eosinophils. Of more concern, however, was the presence of dilated central lacteals seen within some, but not all, of the villi (green arrows). There is also villous atrophy with some fusion of villi. If only endoscopic biopsies had been submitted in this case, a definitive diagnosis would have been difficult to impossible to reach, although the central lacteal dilation would certainly have raised concern. (b) Luckily in this particular case, full-thickness surgical biopsies were submitted. The most striking histological features were present in this low-power view of the outer layers of the intestine (that is, the muscularis and serosa), where we can see multiple, often large lakes of pale-staining eosinophilic material, in some places associated with foamy macrophages (granulomatous or lipogranulomatous inflammation) and early mineralization; this is likely to represent lipogranulomatous lymphadentitis.

Neoplasms

Some neoplasms may only be diagnosed on full-thickness biopsies, in particular those located within the outer layers of the intestines, including smooth muscle tumours (leiomyoma, leiomyosarcoma) and gastrointestinal stromal tumours (GIST). Other tumours may be more reliably diagnosed on full-thickness biopsies. This includes some adenocarcinomas that may be poorly represented in endoscopic biopsies; such biopsies may potentially only capture the more superficial secondary changes such as ulceration, inflammation and necrosis within the mucosa, with the main neoplastic lesion predominantly located in the underlying tissues being easily missed at sampling. Such tumours may not even present as a gross mass, but rather a stenosis of the lumen or a change in thickness of the intestinal wall with loss of layering (Figure 4.6).

Differentiating between severe, diffuse lymphocytic enteritis and small cell, low-grade alimentary lymphoma (LGAL) in cats can be difficult to impossible, particularly in biopsies comprised of mucosa only. Mucosal T-cell lymphoma, which closely matches enteropathy-associated T-cell lymphoma (EATCL) type II (according to the World Health Organization's international classification of tumours of haematopoietic and lymphoid tissues), is most difficult to distinguish from diffuse lymphocytic enteritis. One feature that favours a neoplastic process rather than an inflammatory one is the extension of these small lymphoid cells beyond the mucosa into the submucosa and further, but this feature cannot be assessed in endoscopic samples. This transmural involvement is also important in terms of classification and carries prognostic significance. More on feline LGAL later.

Submitting GI biopsy samples

Histopathological findings in gastric and intestinal biopsies should always be interpreted in conjunction with the clinical history and signalment for any given case. Pertinent clinical history details include species, breed, age, symptoms, duration and any previous and/or current treatments, plus any clinical response to those treatments. Descriptions should be included of any gross changes seen either during exploratory laparotomy or endoscopy. Particularly in the case of endoscopic evaluation, it is best to submit as many samples as possible, and the clinician should always 'take something' in cases where GI disease is suspected or needs to be ruled out, even if no gross lesions are seen at the time of examination (either surgically or endoscopically).

Indicating which level of the GI tract the samples were obtained from is also very important, particularly with endoscopic biopsies; depending on the extent of any pathological changes present, it can sometimes be difficult to determine the site based on the histological appearance alone. Placing samples taken from different levels within the GI tract into separate (labelled) formalin-filled sample pots also allows the pathologist to provide specific results for each individual site or level.

Placing endoscopic biopsies within a 'cell-safe' biopsy insert or capsule and then into the sample pots is also ideal, as it means any particularly small, friable or fragmented samples are not 'lost' within the debris in the bottom of the sample pot; it also reduces the need for histology technicians to further handle the tissues, thereby decreasing the risk of introducing crush artefact at a later stage. Cell-safes can pop open however, so placing each into a separate labelled pot is still necessary.

Interpretation of inflammatory lesions – WSAVA guidelines

So, how does the pathologist assess biopsy samples from inflammatory GI lesions? An initial assessment of the biopsy quantity and type, size and quality will be made first before any further assessment –

Case study 2

A 9-year-old, female (neutered) crossbreed dog presented with a partial obstruction of the intestines. On exploratory laparotomy, there was a focal area of stenosis which was resected and submitted for assessment. Grossly, there was no distinct mass seen, but representative sections were trimmed in for further histological assessment.

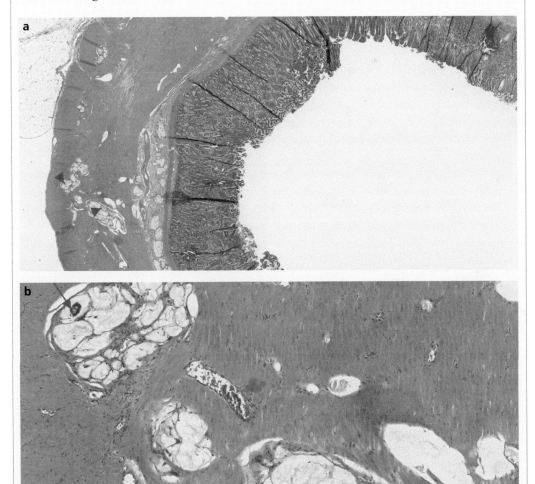

Figure 4.6 (a) In this low-power view, the mucosa, submucosa and muscular layers of the intestine can be seen, as well as adjacent mesenteric adipose tissues. The red arrow heads point to where neoplastic cells can be seen, located within the muscular layer of the wall and associated with lakes of mucinous material. (b) In this higher power view, the red arrows highlight the relatively small number of neoplastic cells actually present, consistent with an intestinal carcinoma.

comments regarding the presence of any crush artefact, fragmentation and the depth of samples aim to reflect how diagnostically useful the samples, and hence the histological findings, are likely to be. This hopefully provides useful feedback to the clinicians in terms of how adequate the biopsies are and whether there may be limitations to the histological assessment.

The World Small Animal Veterinary Association (WSAVA) guidelines for endoscopic GI biopsies from the dog and cat were first published in 2008 and the intention behind the guidelines was to standardize the criteria by which such biopsies are examined; the majority of pathologists now routinely use these guidelines when reporting on GI biopsies. More recently another publication in 2019 modified the system further, but only for dogs.

There are four sets of criteria, each designed for different levels of the GI tract, including the gastric antrum, gastric body, duodenum (but routinely used for all levels of the small intestine) and the colon. For each individual criterion there is a range of 'scores' from normal (0) through mild (1), moderate (2) to severe (3), based on the histological features present.

The histopathological changes are evaluated as follows.

- Surface epithelial (stomach) and villous epithelial (small intestinal) injury; this may vary from attenuation, degeneration, vacuolation or separation of focal areas to more widespread ulceration, depending on the severity.
- Gastric pit epithelial injury (similar to above, stomach).
- Epithelial hyperplasia of gastric pit epithelium, with dilation of gastric pit lumina (gastric antrum).
- Mucosal atrophy – glands (stomach) or crypts (small intestines) separated by a variable amount of fibrous tissues, becoming atrophic, nested and sparse as the severity increases.
- Intra-epithelial lymphocytes in increasing numbers (note there is variation in the normal numbers present in different locations and also between species).
- Lamina propria inflammatory cells; lymphocytes and plasma cells, eosinophils, neutrophils in increasing numbers (again there is variation in normal numbers present in different locations and species). Macrophages would also be assessed within large intestinal biopsies.
- Lymphofollicular hyperplasia in the stomach.
- Villous stunting (small intestines) – evident as variation in width and length, fusion, or blunting.
- Crypt distension (small and large intestines) – presenting as dilation, distortion and/or crypt abscess formation.
- Lacteal dilation (small intestines) – dilation of central lacteal to varying degrees, oedema (for example, as seen in lymphangiectasia).
- Mucosal goblet cells (large intestines) – decreased in number (new addition in 2019).
- Crypt hyperplasia (large intestines).

There are some features not included within the WSAVA guidelines, but which may be commented on by the pathologist. These include the presence or absence of *Helicobacter*-like organisms and other potential pathogens, for example, or loss of crypts (so-called 'crypt drop-out') and crypt epithelial necrosis or regeneration. Owing to the guidelines being designed for endoscopic biopsies rather than full-thickness samples, they also do not include any recommendations for assessment of the outer layers such as the serosa, muscularis or submucosa.

The WSAVA guidelines have some other limitations. One of these is the apparently wide range of 'normal' values for things such as numbers of intra-epithelial lymphocytes and inflammatory cell populations within the lamina propria. There is an overall lack of consensus about what constitutes normal histology in the GI tract, while allowing for any potential differences in 'normal' between different breeds, age groups, different lifestyles and diets. This can make it challenging to identify which cases are definitely abnormal and then to decide which changes have any functional and/or clinical significance. This is further compounded by divergent opinions about the significance of some lesions as well as about the degree of lesion severity between pathologists, despite the introduction of a template via the WSAVA guidelines. Because of the uncertainty over precisely how many leucocytes should be present in the normal GI tract, many pathologists will place much greater weight on any morphological and/or structural changes seen, such as villous atrophy, villous fusion and dysplastic crypts, than on the presence of inflammation, unless the inflammation is moderate or even marked.

The GI tract also has a somewhat limited spectrum of histologic responses to an inflammatory process, regardless of the underlying aetiology. So even if significant changes are present, the pathologist can often only provide a morphological diagnosis, that is, a diagnosis based on the predominant changes seen in the tissues together with a list of potential causes, rather than a specific diagnosis, cause or disease.

Luminal contents are also examined for the presence of any possible pathogens – including bacteria (such as *Helicobacter*-like organisms), as well as protozoans (including *Giardia*, *Tritrichomonas* and *Cryptosporidium* species, as well as coccidia), fungi, and nematodes and other helminths. The presence of organisms within histological sections does not necessarily signify clinical significance, however. For example, the precise role of *Helicobacter* infection in gastric disease remains somewhat uncertain – given this, most pathologists will simply report on their presence, approximate numbers (low, medium or high) and their location (that is, if they are present deep within the gastric pits or overlying the mucosal surface) rather than directly ascribing any concurrent inflammation to their presence (Figure 4.7). Aetiological diagnoses are not often made on either endoscopic or full-thickness biopsies. This is probably for a

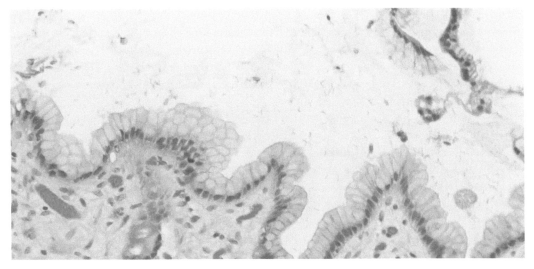

Figure 4.7 Medium power overview showing moderate numbers of *Helicobacter*-like organisms overlying the mucosal surface, within a gastric biopsy from a dog.

number of reasons: histology is not a particularly sensitive technique for detecting many of these agents; and/or they may not necessarily produce aetiologically specific histological changes.

Another source of frustration for clinicians (and pathologists) is the apparent lack of correlation between the severity of histological changes and the presenting clinical signs. Multiple studies have failed to identify any strong association between clinical findings and histopathological lesions in dogs with enteritis even when post-treatment improvements in clinical signs were compared to the post-treatment histological appearance, although there is some evidence that dogs with moderate to severe enteritis are more likely to have histological changes than those dogs presenting with only mild clinical signs.

What we cannot tell you

Some GI diseases simply cannot be diagnosed by light microscopy, regardless of sample thickness, either because they are functional diseases (for example, ileus) or because the defect is ultrastructural in nature (for example, brush border abnormalities). Such conditions require additional techniques (such as electron microscopy in the case of ultrastructural lesions) to identify them.

Feline intestinal lymphoma, IHC and PARR

Feline low grade alimentary lymphoma (LGAL) is sometimes referred to as small cell lymphoma, or diffuse low-grade lymphoma, and considered equivalent to EATCL type II in people. For histopathologists, it can be really difficult or sometimes even impossible to differentiate between LGAL and a severe, predominantly lymphocytic enteritis, because for both of these diseases, the cells involved are predominantly small lymphocytes. There are very few mitotic figures in LGAL because it is 'low grade'.

Starting with the HE sections, there are some additional features pathologists look for in addition to the small lymphocytes, and finding some or any of these may increase our index of suspicion for lymphoma. These include increased numbers of lymphocytes within the villous epithelial layer (and the crypt epithelium, that is, the intra-epithelial lymphocytes). Sometimes these lymphocytes may form nests, plaques and clusters, and they even begin to obscure the boundary between the lamina propria and the epithelial layer (Figure 4.8). Other features for concern would include obliteration of the normal structures such as the crypts, an absence of other inflammatory cell types, the presence of any mitotic figures, and any evidence of extension of the small lymphocytes beyond the mucosal layer and into the submucosa and beyond (obviously we cannot assess this in endoscopic biopsies). Some of these features can be incredibly focal, affecting just a few villi, or even just parts of villi, so the pathologist must carefully examine all of the tissues on the slide.

The situation is further complicated in some instances by the presence of both conditions within the same individual, or the fact that some cats appear to initially present with enteritis but subsequently develop LGAL at a later stage. I do not think we currently fully understand these conditions in cats, and whether this represents progression over time from an enteritis to LGAL, or whether the LGAL was always present but was missed before. More recently there have been several publications which appear to diagnose LGAL (including the use of IHC and PARR) in clinically normal cats, which further muddies the water!

In cases such as this, I personally like to take a stepwise approach to the diagnosis, as proposed by Kiupel et al. in 2011. The first step is the histopathology, preferably in correlation with the clinical signs. Does it look inflammatory on the initial HE sections? If it does, treat accordingly. Does it respond as expected? If no, then reconsider the diagnosis!

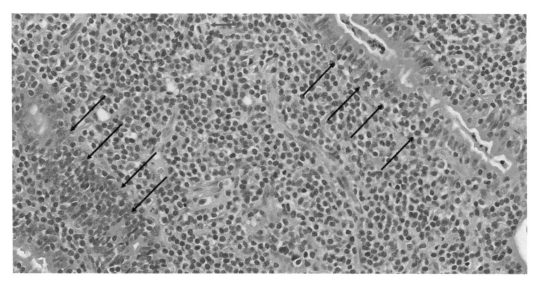

Figure 4.8 A high-power view of an intestinal biopsy from a cat with possible LGAL. Dark blue arrows are indicating small lymphocytes infiltrating into crypt epithelium in large numbers; although they are not forming clusters or nests, they are beginning to obscure the boundary between epithelium and lamina propria. The red arrow indicates a mitotic figure within a small lymphocyte. The red oval indicates there are also small numbers of plasma cells present, so the cellular infiltrate is slightly mixed. This cat subsequently had LGAL confirmed via IHC and PARR testing.

If on the initial HE sections lymphoma is suspected, then the next step is to perform immunohisto-chemistry (IHC), to ascertain whether the lymphocytes present are all T-cells, all B-cells or a mixture of both. If they are all the same immunophenotype, this supports a diagnosis of lymphoma. If they are a mixture of B-cells and T-cells, then it is more suggestive of an inflammatory process. If these lympho-cytes are all the same type, then the IHC also tells you the immunophenotype of the lymphoma. LGAL are T-cell lymphomas.

If the diagnosis remains uncertain, then the next step is to progress to PARR testing. As described in more detail later in this book, PARR is a PCR-based assay looking for evidence of clonal expansion within the lymphocyte population. If the lymphocytes present are all the same clone this means they all have the same rearrangement of their T-cell (or B-cell) receptor, which would suggest they have all arisen from one individual cell, that is, that this is a neoplastic cell population. If there is a mixture present, this means there are lots of different clones which have expanded to produce the lymphocyte population seen, and this is more suggestive of an inflammatory response. At each step, the pathologist and clinician are add-ing this information to the clinical picture and correlating it with any clinical response to therapy. These results, IHC and PARR, are not intended to be interpreted in isolation.

A polite plea on behalf of pathologists, please do not be tempted to skip the IHC (or even the HE) and go straight for PARR testing. There are several reasons for this over and above the fact that without the HE and IHC findings, you are missing potentially vital parts of the puzzle. Technically speaking, you cannot immunophenotype a lymphoma with 100% confidence based on PARR alone, because these are neoplastic cells and they do not follow the rules! They can be immunophenotypically T-cells (for example) and yet demonstrate a clonal rearrangement in the B-cell receptor (and vice versa). Although PARR will give you an indication of T-cell or B-cell, in a minority of cases this will be misleading – although you will not know which cases these are.

PARR is not a perfect test and there is the potential for both false positive and false negative results; these are more easily detected when the results are interpreted in conjunction with other clinical and histological findings. This is particularly the case in cats, as we do not yet have as detailed a knowledge of the TCR (T-cell receptor) and BCR (B-cell receptor) regions and their potential variations – and hence we do not yet have the best primers to use in the PCR reactions, and we are probably not covering all the potential gene rearrangements. And then there are in-between results where you have a low number of clones (oligoclonal) – how do we interpret those? We wonder whether some immune-mediated diseases might fall into this category, or some infectious diseases, because a restricted subset of clones are expanding, but as yet we simply do not know.

Liver biopsies

Pros and cons of Tru-cut versus surgical biopsies

Of course, as the saying goes, the more tissue you give the pathologist, the happier they are; so, while wedge biopsies are preferred, we of course realize these may not be practical or safe to perform in all cases. Tru-cut biopsies from the liver are becoming more common submissions to the laboratory, but it is important to realize their limitations, and to help understand this a quick revision of the lobular architecture of the liver is helpful (Figure 4.9). Remember that each lobule has a central vein surrounded by radiating cords

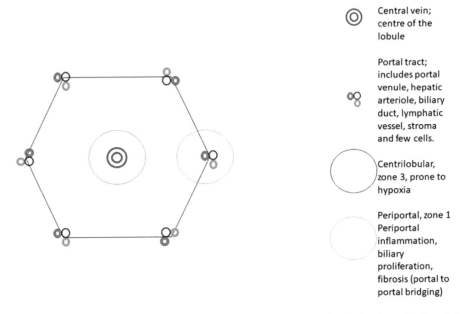

Central vein; centre of the lobule

Portal tract; includes portal venule, hepatic arteriole, biliary duct, lymphatic vessel, stroma and few cells.

Centrilobular, zone 3, prone to hypoxia

Periportal, zone 1 Periportal inflammation, biliary proliferation, fibrosis (portal to portal bridging)

Figure 4.9 Schematic illustration of a hepatic lobule, with the central vein in the middle of the lobule surrounded by radiating cords of hepatocytes and sinusoids. At the periphery are the portal tracts, which contain portal venules, hepatic arterioles, biliary ducts, lymphatic vessels and occasional cells within a small amount of stroma.

a

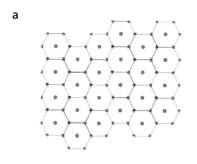

b

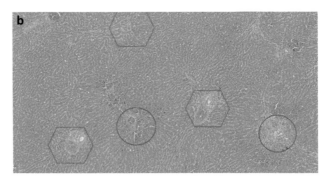

Figure 4.10 (a) Schematic representation of a wedge biopsy from the liver, showing the arrangement of lobules adjacent to one another, with common portal tracts. Such a biopsy will allow assessment of the overall lobular architecture, the distribution of any pathological changes (including necrosis/degeneration of hepatocytes, inflammation, fibrosis) and also the assessment of a larger numbers of portal tracts. (b) Wedge biopsy from the liver of a dog, at low-power, showing the lobular architecture. The red circle is a central vein, and the blue hexagons are the surrounding portal tracts.

a   b

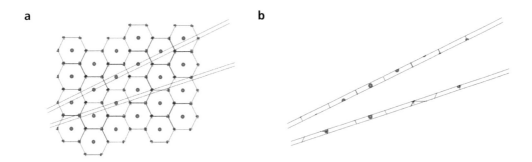

Figure 4.11 (a, b) Schematic representation of Tru-cut needle biopsies from the same part of the liver as shown in Figure 4.10a. Note that only a very small number of sometimes incomplete portal tracts are available for assessment, and that the lobular architecture cannot be reliably examined. Focal lesions may or may not be present.

of hepatocytes separated by sinusoids, with multiple portal tracts at the periphery. Portal tracts include portal venules, hepatic arterioles, lymphatic vessels, some stroma and occasional cells such as lymphocytes.

Now imagine multiple lobules arranged in a pattern similar to that illustrated in Figure 4.10a – this is a schematic representation of what a pathologist would see when assessing a wedge biopsy from the liver – whereas Figure 4.11 illustrates what a pathologist might see when only Tru-cut biopsies are submitted from the same part of the liver.

For comparison, in human medicine, a minimum of 11–15 complete portal tracts are required to adequately assess the liver for diffuse conditions, but from personal experience it is uncommon for this number of portal tracts to be present within liver Tru-cut biopsy submissions from our veterinary patients. The adequacy of any particular form of biopsy is also somewhat dependent on the disease

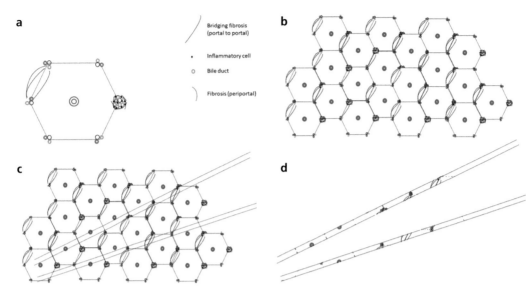

Figure 4.12 (a) Schematic representation of an 'abnormal liver lobule' – in this case some changes are periportal, including biliary hyperplasia, periportal inflammation and fibrosis. There is also some portal-to-portal bridging fibrosis. Such changes may not affect all lobules / periportal areas equally. (b) Schematic representation of a wedge biopsy from the liver with changes affecting some portal tracts, as above. Such a biopsy would allow for assessment of abnormal portal tracts, and also the extent of any fibrosis, including bridging fibrosis – this is where fibrosis extends between adjacent portal tracts and/or between adjacent central veins, depending on the pattern of fibrosis present. (c and d) Schematic representation of Tru-cut needle biopsies from the same part of the 'abnormal' liver. Only a very small number of sometimes incomplete but abnormal portal tracts are present, as are the areas of fibrosis, but the distribution of the fibrosis and whether it is bridging adjacent portal areas cannot be readily determined.

process or processes present, so the clinical differential diagnosis list will play an important role in deciding which form of biopsy to take. If the process is diffuse throughout part or all of the organ, then a small biopsy will most likely contain a representative portion. However, if the lesion is focal or multifocal then there is the possibility of missing it, or of it being poorly represented. A problem also arises if the pathological processes vary between fields, for example in cirrhosis where there are areas of fibrosis and nodular regeneration, a biopsy may well only include regenerative tissues potentially resulting in a misleading diagnosis, or a less definitive list of differential diagnoses, in the best-case scenario.

Differentiation between some nodular lesions depends on assessment of this lobular architecture, which is more difficult in Tru-cut biopsy samples. An example would be distinguishing between nodular hyperplasia where lobular architecture and portal tracts should still be present although distorted, or a well-differentiated hepatocellular tumour (benign or low-grade malignant) where the key feature is often the absence of portal tracts – thus a pathologist faced with Tru-cut biopsies from a nodular liver with cords of hepatocytes but no portal tracts may struggle to differentiate between nodular hyperplasia and a hepatocellular neoplasm.

Some changes have different distributions within the liver (whole or contiguous lobules – Figure 4.12a) and the pattern of distribution can often provide useful indications as to underlying causes; again, assessment of this distribution is more challenging with Tru-cut biopsies (Figure 4.12c and d) versus wedge biopsy (Figure 4.12b). For example, with hepatocyte degeneration and/or necrosis a centrilobular pattern is often associated with hypoxia as the underlying cause, due to severe anaemia or right-sided heart failure, and a periportal pattern is uncommon but may occur following exposure to certain toxins (a midzonal pattern is rare and often toxin-associated). The nature and distribution of inflammatory lesions in the liver are often dictated by the route of entry, the host response and the nature of any infectious agent involved. For example, a haematogenous route tends to cause a random multifocal distribution of lesions – this includes bacterial or metastatic tumour emboli. Infections that ascend the biliary tract are typically centred on bile ducts, although severe lesions may affect the entire portal tract and extend into the adjacent parenchyma.

Other important changes will be seen within portal tracts, for example biliary hyperplasia, which particularly occurs in diseases that obstruct normal bile drainage. An absence of portal veins and increased numbers of small calibre arterioles can be seen in congenital portosystemic shunts. Portal tracts may also be the site of fibrosis; the distribution and severity of fibrosis can be indicative of the type of insult and is of prognostic significance, but assessment is hampered if lobular architecture cannot be examined. Bridging fibrosis is of particular concern as disruption of the normal hepatic structure will impair liver function.

How does the pathologist assess a liver biopsy?

As with any tissue or organ, it is important that the pathologist has a consistent and systematic approach. This may vary between pathologists, however. Below is my own approach to a liver biopsy.

Quality check

- What amount of tissue is available?
- What is the nature of biopsy (Tru-cut or wedge)?
- If Tru-cut, how many/what length/how many portal tracts are there?
- Are there any artefact, fixation issues and so on that will hamper my assessment?
- Do I need further sections or special stains to help my interpretation?
- Is it diagnostic? Maybe it is all necrotic, or haemorrhagic. Sometimes Tru-cut biopsies have a lot of muscle and connective tissues present as well.

Then at low power, is there a mass or masses present?

- What is their distribution within the samples and in relation to the lobular structure?

This may tell us something about the spread or route of involvement; for example, a periportal process could be ascending from the biliary, or a random distribution scattered throughout might be embolic spread (neoplasia, infectious via haematogenous spread).

Then, still at low power, an assessment of *the overall lobular architecture*.

- Are there lobules present, with portal tracts, central veins and so on?
- Are the lobules all similar in size or are they uneven? Are some portal tracts closer together than others?

- Is the capsular surface undulating? These things will suggest something has been added or is absent.
- Is the capsular surface covered by anything (fibrin, neutrophils, reactive mesothelial cells)? This might tell us something about what is going on outside of the liver.
- Is there anything in the liver that should not be there, or anything that should be that is not? (The second is actually harder for pathologists to spot!)

Assessment of the portal tracts

- Do any of the portal tracts look variable in size?
- Are they expanded – if so by how much?
- Are they lacking anything – for example, in some vascular anomalies?
- Are they expanded by fibrosis? Special staining for collagen helps to highlight this and show where it is. Is it in the portal areas or starting to expand into the surrounding parenchyma? Is the fibrosis bridging? Portal to portal?
- Is there biliary hyperplasia?
- Are there dilated vessels?
- Are there any inflammatory cells, what type, how many, where are they?
- Are there any neoplastic cells, what type?

Assessment of hepatocytes

- Any vacuolation, or necrosis (single cell or focal areas, distribution)?
- Any evidence of regeneration (anisokaryosis, bi-nucleate cells, mitotic activity)?
- Pigment accumulation, what type? Special stains that can help differentiate between some of these pigments, like copper, haemosiderin and bile (see Chapter 5).
- Distribution – which cells are affected/number affected? Is a particular zone of the lobule more affected than others?

Sinusoids

- Is there any evidence of dilation, congestion, inflammatory cells, amyloidosis or haemorrhage affecting the sinusoids?
- Are the Kupffer cells within sinusoids showing any changes?

If inflammatory, is this a reactive hepatopathy or a true hepatitis?

Webster et al.'s (2019) 'ACVIM consensus statement on the diagnosis and treatment of chronic hepatitis in dogs' is extremely useful, and helps us to divide liver biopsies with inflammatory disease into three broad categories, namely lobular dissecting hepatitis, primary chronic hepatitis or secondary non-specific reactive hepatopathy. The distinction also incorporates the clinical scenario also, so again it is important for this clinical information to be made available to the pathologist.

Distinction between primary inflammatory hepatopathies and secondary or reactive hepatopathy is an important one; a secondary or reactive hepatopathy is a response by the liver to a process occurring elsewhere, and the inflammation seen in the liver is not accompanied by any fibrosis or hepatocyte necrosis/apoptosis. This finding should prompt the clinician to look for an extra-hepatic disorder, such as an endocrinopathy or an enteritis. Think of the liver as a giant lymph node, sieving through all of the blood supply from the GI tract.

A primary hepatopathy can then be further characterized by a number of features, as previously described. These include the presence, severity, location and nature of any inflammatory cell infiltrate present, the presence of any hepatocyte degeneration/regeneration/necrosis/apoptosis (distribution, severity), the presence of any fibrosis (distribution, and whether there is any portal–portal or portal–central bridging with subsequent architectural distortion), any regenerative nodules, biliary proliferation, and pigment accumulation.

Fibrosis is a key feature and is a hallmark of chronicity. It often starts as expansion of portal tracts and progresses over time into thicker or broader bands of fibrous stroma, eventually extending between adjacent portal areas (portal–portal bridging) or between portal areas of central veins (portal–central bridging). At this stage, the term cirrhosis may begin to be used – typically when bridging fibrosis is seen in conjunction with regenerative nodules. Bridging fibrosis is of concern because by this stage there is marked disruption of the normal lobular architecture, which will in turn impair hepatic function.

Copper and canine chronic hepatopathy

Copper accumulates in the liver of dogs with chronic hepatopathies and can be seen as a primary cause (primary copper associated hepatopathy) evident in a growing number of breeds. However, it is also seen accumulating secondary to other causes of hepatopathy. Therefore, the finding of copper in and of itself is not diagnostic for a primary copper associated hepatopathy. There is a difference in the quantity and distribution of copper accumulation seen in primary copper associated hepatopathy as opposed to secondary, but in my experience, it can be sometimes difficult to confidently distinguish between the two, particularly if other changes to the hepatic parenchyma are also severe and distort the lobular architecture and/or in Tru-cut biopsies with few intact lobules. It is very important to assess for the presence of copper, as chelating agents are a potential therapeutic option, regardless of whether the accumulation is primary or secondary.

Special staining for copper (typically with stains such as rhodanine, or rubeanic acid) is typically performed on canine liver biopsies for this reason. These special stains detect the presence of copper, the distribution (periportal versus centrilobular), and can allow for a subjective assessment of the severity of any such accumulation. Assessment also entails identifying which cells are accumulating the copper (macrophages and/or hepatocytes) and whether its presence is associated with necrotic hepatocytes, and formation of small 'copper granulomas'.

More precise quantification requires analysis of tissues (fresh or formalin-fixed tissue is acceptable, but not formalin-fixed, paraffin-embedded) – there are various different techniques available which require differing amounts of liver tissue. Note, however, that the amount of copper can vary between different lobes of the liver, so some care is required in interpretation, and you may need to consider sampling from multiple lobes. There may also appear to be a discrepancy between histological findings and copper quantification for this very same reason, so it is important to note where samples are obtained from.

Self-assessment: multiple choice questions

An 11-year-old, female (neutered) domestic short hair cat with a long history of intermittent vomiting and inappetence has now presented to your clinic with diarrhoea and progressive weight loss. The owner agrees to GI endoscopy and biopsy as part of investigation.

1. When submitting the endoscopic GI biopsies:
    a   you should include a clinical history and signalment, including the symptoms, their duration and any previous and/or current treatments and any clinical response to those treatments
    b   place samples from each level of the GI tract in a cell-safe, and then into an individual, labelled sample pot
    c   remember that only the mucosa will be available for assessment by the pathologist and this may limit what information can be gained from the biopsies
    d   all of the above are true.
2. Samples from the small intestines show a diffuse infiltrate predominantly composed of small lymphocytes. What features present on the HE sections might raise concern for a low-grade alimentary lymphoma?
    a   plasma cells admixed with the lymphocytes
    b   villi which are equal in width and length, with no evidence of villous blunting or fusion
    c   increased numbers of intra-epithelial lymphocytes which obscure the interface between the epithelial layer and the lamina propria
    d   infiltrates confined to the mucosal layer
3. What additional testing might you consider to confirm or exclude the potential differential diagnosis of low-grade alimentary lymphoma? (There is more than one correct answer here!)
    a   immunohistochemical (IHC) staining for B-lymphocytes and T-lymphocytes
    b   PARR testing for clonality, no need for IHC
    c   immunohistochemical staining for B-lymphocytes and T-lymphocytes, followed by PARR testing if the infiltrate is predominantly T-cell on IHC and further confirmation is wanted
    d   special staining for bacteria
4. Which of the following structures are NOT present in portal tracts of the liver?
    a   biliary ducts
    b   hepatocytes
    c   portal venules
    d   hepatic arterioles
5. How many complete portal tracts are required to adequately assess the liver for diffuse conditions in human medicine?
    a   11–15
    b   1–5
    c   25
    d   50
6. Which of the following special stains is used to detect the presence of copper in liver biopsies?
    a   Perls
    b   Masson's trichrome

   c Fouchet

   d Rhodanine

7. The presence of which of the following features in liver biopsies from a dog would suggest a secondary or reactive hepatopathy rather than a primary inflammatory hepatopathy?

   a hepatocyte necrosis

   b fibrosis

   c inflammatory cells in sinusoids

   d hepatocyte apoptosis

The answers are available on page 174.

5

Special stains, immunohistochemistry and additional testing

Introduction

This chapter provides an overview of the most commonly used special stains and when and why they might be requested. There is then an explanation of how immunohistochemistry works and an introduction to some of the more commonly used 'markers', along with a discussion of how and when these may be used for the identification of infectious agents, tumour differentiation/diagnosis and also increasingly for prognostication. There is also a brief section on some other molecular tests pathologists most frequently request on cases, particularly PARR testing for lymphoma, and in situ hybridization (ISH) for identifying infectious agents.

Special stains

This section summarizes the most commonly used 'special stains' utilized in a diagnostic setting, their indications and the clinical situations where they might be useful. The HE stain is the routine, everyday stain used in histological sections and will typically be the first slide a pathologist looks at for any given case (Figure 5.1). Haematoxylin colours nuclei and a few other objects blue (referred to as 'basophilic'), while the eosin counterstains the cytoplasm in various shades of pink (termed 'pale' to 'brightly' to 'deeply eosinophilic' depending on the precise shade). Structures do not have to be acidic or basic to

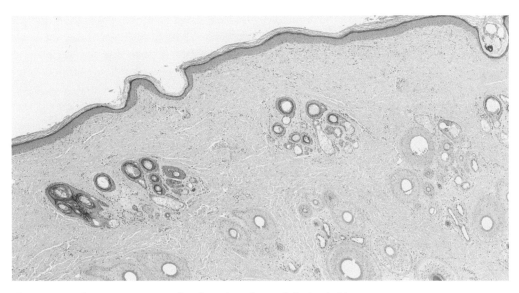

Figure 5.1 A low-power HE stained section through haired skin.

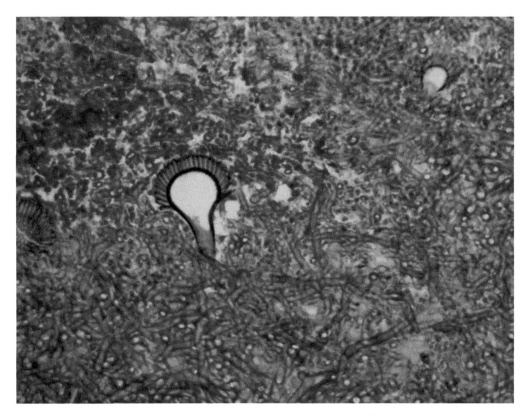

Figure 5.2 A higher power HE stained section through a fungal plaque, with naturally pigmented fungal hyphae (cultured as *Aspergillus*).

be called basophilic or eosinophilic, the terminology is simply based on the affinity to the dyes. There is some variation in HE stains between different laboratories, with some appearing more pink or blue than others. Other, endogenous colours may also be present in a histology section, for example erythrocytes are bright red, melanin is brown-black and other pigments may be yellow, golden-brown or green (Figure 5.2).

Based on the appearance of an initial HE section, a pathologist may request further 'special' stains for a number of reasons. Some particular tissue structures do not stain well with routine HE staining. For example, the reticular fibres in the liver require a silver stain such as Gordon-Sweets to allow better assessment of liver architecture, while Masson's trichrome stains connective tissues, highlighting the presence of fibrosis in cases of liver and heart disease (Figure 5.3). Hydrophobic structures also tend to remain clear since these are usually rich in fats; this includes adipocytes and the myelin around neuron axons. Some special stains aid better identification of poorly differentiated neoplastic cells (for example, mast cells or a mucin-secreting neoplasia), or may highlight the presence of infectious agents. Other stains allow more precise identification of deposits such as amyloid, calcium and a variety of pigments.

This section is not intended as an exhaustive list of special stains, as there are a very large number of them; it will instead concentrate on the ones most often used in routine histopathology cases and why they might be used.

Metachromatic stains

Metachromatic stains are those which have the ability to produce different colours with various histologic or cytologic structures. The most well-known examples include Giemsa, Wright and Diff-Quick stains. The Giemsa stain has multiple purposes within diagnostics; it is one of the classic stains used for peripheral blood smears and bone marrow specimens, and is also useful for staining some fungal species and some intracellular protozoa. Another major use of Giemsa, as well as other metachromatic stains such as Toluidine blue and Astra blue, is the identification of mast cells. This is because the Giemsa stain turns the cytoplasmic granules present in mast cells magenta to purple in colour (Figure 5.4a), while the Toluidine blue stains them blue (Figure 5.4b).

These stains may aid better differentiation of a round cell tumour as being of mast cell origin, especially in some of the more poorly differentiated tumours where the granules may not be obvious in the routine HE sections. In other cases, where increased numbers of mast cells are present in a lesion that is otherwise inflammatory in appearance, a Giemsa stain can help reveal just how many mast cells are present, whether they form clusters, how pleomorphic they are, whether they contain mitotic figures and whether the pathologist should be suspicious of an underlying neoplasm. The Giemsa stain can also help when assessing mast cell tumour margins, scar line resections, and also when looking for evidence of metastatic spread to regional lymph nodes. However, it is really important to remember it cannot distinguish between neoplastic mast cells and the non-neoplastic mast cells which are migrating to the site of the tumour, attracted by the release of histamine and other bioactive substances.

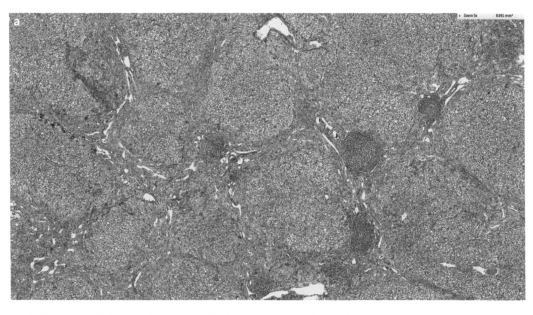

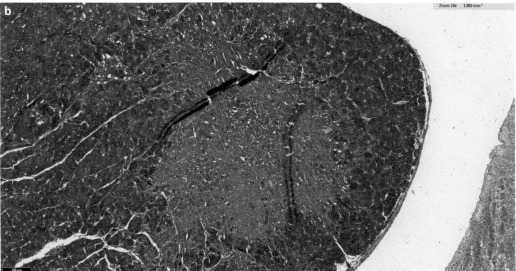

Figure 5.3 Masson's trichrome staining, highlighting the presence of fibrosis (blue): (a) a feline liver biopsy with suspected congenital hepatic fibrosis; (b) replacement fibrosis (scarring) in a section of feline heart, with an underlying cardiomyopathy.

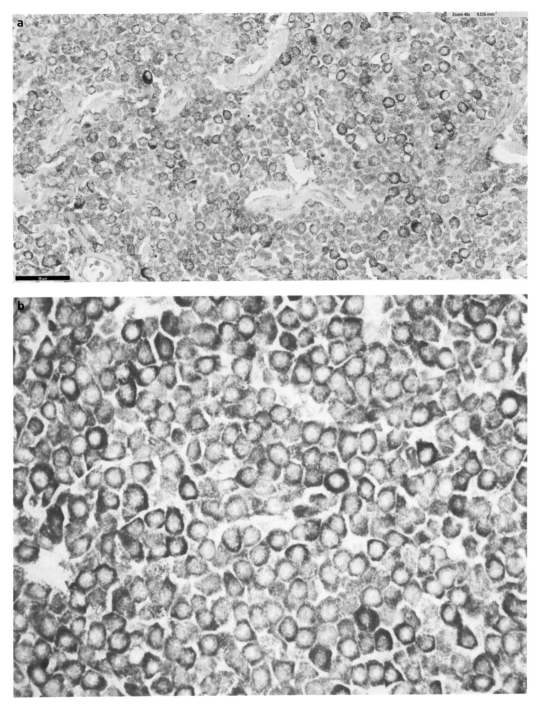

Figure 5.4 Metachromatic staining of mast cell granules: (a) Giemsa staining of a canine mast cell tumour (granules are magenta); (b) Toluidine blue staining of a feline mast cell tumour (granules are blue).

Stains for infectious agents

Gram and Warthin–Starry stains

Gram staining is a method for highlighting the presence and morphology of bacterial populations within a histology section; it also differentiates bacterial species into two large groups, either gram-positive or gram-negative, based on the chemical and physical properties of their cell walls. It detects peptidoglycan, which is present in a thick layer in gram-positive bacteria and results in a blue/purple colour. Gram-negative bacteria generally have a thin layer of peptidoglycan between two membranes, which results in a pink/red colour (Figure 5.5a). Not all bacteria can be definitively classified by this technique, thus there are gram-variable and gram-indeterminate groups as well. Gram-positive bacteria include many well-known genera such as *Bacillus*, *Listeria*, *Staphylococcus*, *Streptococcus*, *Enterococcus* and *Clostridium*, while gram-negative bacteria include *Bordetella*, *Campylobacter*, *Enterobacter*, *Escherichia coli*, *Helicobacter*, *Pasteurella*, *Pseudomonas* and *Salmonella*. Remember, however, that gram staining is not always reliable in histological sections and follow-up culture, full identification and antimicrobial sensitivity testing of any potentially significant bacterial populations seen on histology is always recommended.

Warthin–Starry is a silver-nitrate based staining technique that is used to detect spirochetes such as *Leptospira* and *Borrelia*, as well as *Helicobacter* species which may be present in gastric biopsies (Figure 5.5b).

Ziehl–Neelsen stain

The Ziehl–Neelsen (ZN) stain, also known as the acid-fast stain, is a special stain used to identify acid-fast organisms, mainly Mycobacterial species such as *M. bovis*, *M. paratuberculosis* and *M. avium*. These may be present within suspicious lesions in very low numbers, which means identification on routine HE sections is often nigh-on impossible (Figure 5.6). Specialized cultures or molecular techniques such as PCR are required to confirm the identification of *Mycobacterium* species and to rule out other acid-fast bacilli (although other types of bacilli are extremely unlikely) and also to precisely identify the species of *Mycobacterium* involved. The ZN stain can also be used to identify intranuclear lead inclusion bodies.

Periodic acid-Schiff

Periodic acid-Schiff (PAS) is a staining method used to detect glycogen and other polysaccharides in tissues. Probably the most common use of PAS in diagnostic pathology is for fungal infections (Figure 5.7a), such as *Malassezia*, fungal hyphae and *Candida* (living fungi). Other stains, especially silver stains, are also used to detect fungal organisms, for example Grocott's methenamine silver stain (Figure 5.7b; fungi both dead and alive).

The presence of glycogen can be confirmed in tissue sections by using diastase to digest the glycogen from a section, then comparing a diastase-digested PAS section with a normal PAS section. If the positive-staining material present in the PAS slide is glycogen, then it will be absent from the corresponding location on the diastase-digested slide. This technique can be used on liver sections to confirm intracytoplasmic material is glycogen, as opposed to fat, and can be used on neurological tissues to distinguish glycogen storage diseases from other types of storage disease.

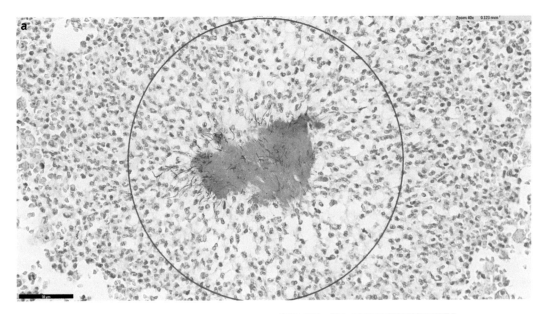

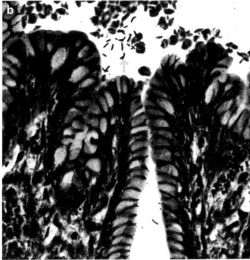

Figure 5.5 (a) Gram stain highlighting the presence of bacteria within an abscess, dog. Gram-positive (blue) filamentous organisms. (b) Warthin–Starry stain highlighting the presence of *Helicobacter*-like organisms (black, arrowed), gastric mucosa, dog.

Congo red stain for amyloid

Amyloid is a fairly homogenous rather nondescript eosinophilic material on routine HE stained sections, and if suspected its presence ideally needs to be confirmed by special stains such as Congo red. This particular stain colours amyloid an orange-red colour, and when viewed under a polarized light the material demonstrates apple-green birefringence. Amyloid may be present within tissues due to a range of disease processes. Primary amyloidosis is the most common systemic or generalized form; most often this is due to plasma cell or B-cell dyscrasias, such as multiple myeloma and other monoclonal B-cell proliferations, resulting in increased amounts of immunoglobulin light chain (AL amyloid), which forms the basis of

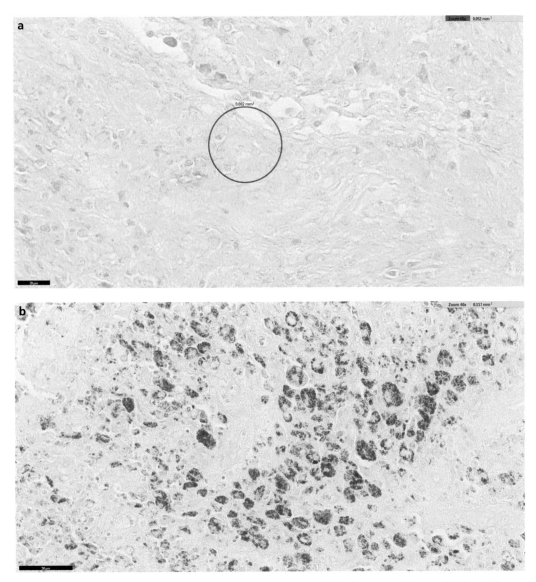

Figure 5.6 Ziehl–Neelsen staining of *Mycobacterium* sp.: (a) lesion containing a single acid-fast organism; (b) lesion containing very large numbers of acid-fast organisms, both cats. Organisms are dark red magenta against the background counterstain which is light blue.

the amyloid present in these cases. Secondary or reactive amyloidosis is when the amyloid is generated from increased amounts of the acute phase protein serum amyloid A (AA amyloid) and is typically associated with chronic inflammatory conditions or neoplasia, although it can also be idiopathic. Familial amyloidosis is a hereditary and systemic condition which can affect various organ systems. It is seen in Abyssinian cats and Shar Pei dogs (Figure 5.8), where deposition occurs in the kidney and in Siamese cats, where it occurs in the liver.

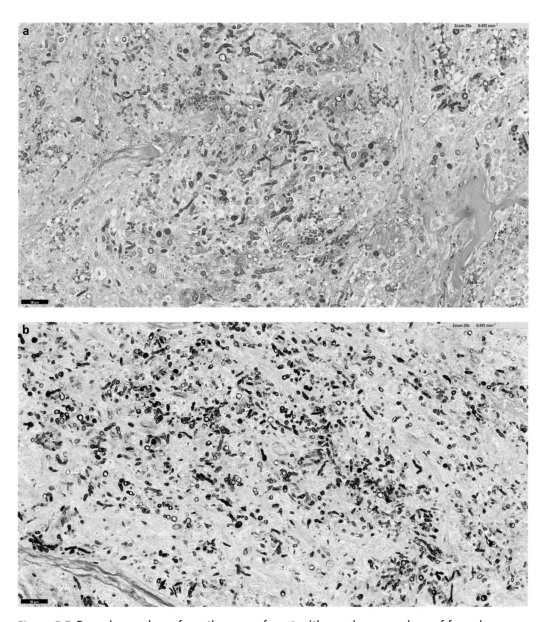

Figure 5.7 Fungal granuloma from the nose of a cat with very large numbers of fungal hyphae, stained with (a) PAS (purple hyphae) or (b) Grocott's (black hyphae).

Von Kossa stain for calcium

The presence of calcium within tissues is confirmed by the von Kossa stain, which colours calcium black. Pathological calcification of tissues falls into two broad categories: dystrophic (serum calcium levels are normal, but the tissue is not); and metastatic (serum calcium levels are increased, but the tissues are normal). Dystrophic calcification can occur in necrotic tissues, such as in the centre of

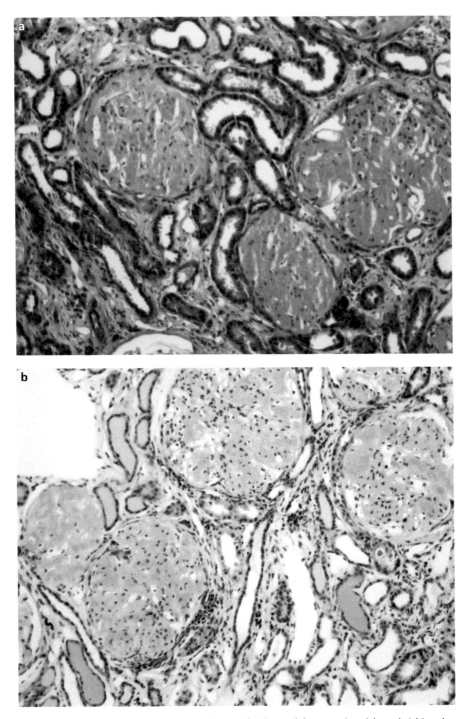

Figure 5.8 Renal biopsy from a Shar Pei with amyloidosis: (a) HE stained (amyloid in glomeruli is pink); (b) Congo red stained (amyloid is orange-red).

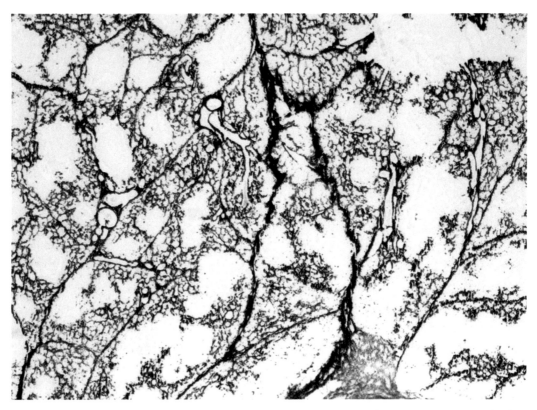

Figure 5.9 Von Kossa stained section of mesenteric adipose tissues, from a puppy which died after having ingested a tube of the owner's Psoriasis cream, causing vitamin D toxicosis and widespread mineralization of tissues throughout the body. Calcium stains black.

granulomas in tuberculosis and Johne's disease. It can also be seen in the skin of dogs, for example, calcinosis cutis associated with hyperadrenocorticism (Cushing's disease) and calcinosis circumscripta (occurring in the skin and other soft tissues) associated with sites of repeated trauma. Metastatic calcification can be seen associated with renal failure (secondary hyperparathyroidism), vitamin D toxicosis (ingestion of calcinogenic plants, rodenticides) (Figure 5.9), primary hyperparathyroidism, pseudohyperparathyroidism (release of parathyroid-related protein from certain tumours) and destructive bone lesions.

Pigment stains

Masson's Fontana

Melanocytic tumours can represent a diagnostic challenge in several ways. Poorly melanized or amelanotic tumours can vary markedly in their cellular morphology, and in the absence of melanin as a clue, they can resemble a large number of other tumours. Masson's Fontana (alternatively known as Masson–Fontana or Fontana–Masson) is a stain that detects melanin pigment and which aids diagnosis in poorly melanized tumours by highlighting the presence of any small amounts of melanin (Figure 5.10),

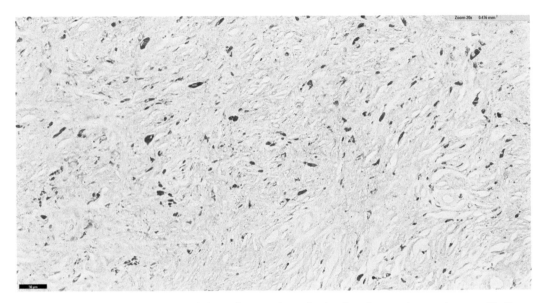

Figure 5.10 Masson's Fontana staining of a poorly melanized melanocytic neoplasm, with the melanin pigment staining brown-black.

and allows distinction between melanin and any other similar pigments which may be present, such as haemosiderin.

Permanganate bleach

Large amounts of melanin pigment within the tumour cells can obscure both nuclear and cellular morphology, making histological assessment of malignancy difficult. Bleaching of sections with permanganate bleach removes the colour of the pigment and allows clearer assessment of nuclear morphology and the mitotic count, important features for distinguishing between malignant or benign tumours.

Other pigment stains

Various stains are available to help the pathologist distinguish between different pigments present in histological sections. For example, the Dunn–Thompson stain for haemoglobin may be of use in cases of intravascular haemolysis leading to deposition of haemoglobin within renal tubules. The Fouchet stain (Figure 5.11) for bile pigments may be used in cases of cholestasis. Perl's Prussian blue is used to highlight the presence of haemosiderin, and to distinguish it from other pigments (Figure 5.12). Examples include the presence of haemosiderin within alveolar macrophages seen with passive chronic congestion of the lungs (so-called 'heart-failure cells'). Copper granules in canine hepatopathy cases can be highlighted and confirmed by stains such as Rhodanine (Figure 5.13) and Rubeanic acid.

Fat stains

Various stains are used to detect the presence of fat in a section. However, they require the use of frozen tissue sections, which not all laboratories have the facilities to offer. Normal routine processing of tissues

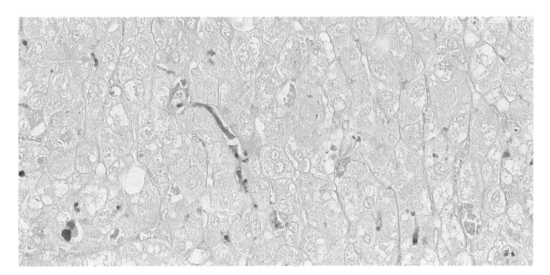

Figure 5.11 Fouchet stain for bile (emerald green) on a liver biopsy from a dog, showing bile plugging (arrowed in green).

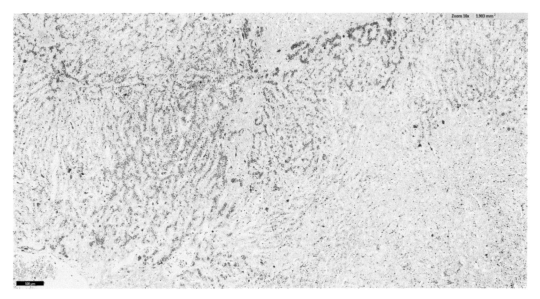

Figure 5.12 Perl's Prussian blue staining of a canine liver biopsy, with large amounts of haemosiderin present (blue).

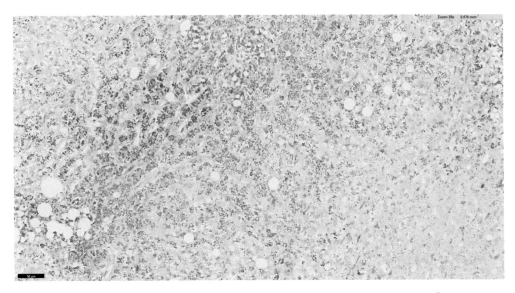

Figure 5.13 Rhodanine staining of a canine liver biopsy, with large amounts of copper present (red brown).

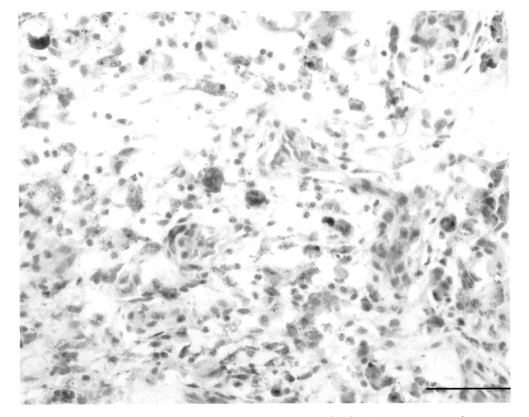

Figure 5.14 Oil red O staining on a frozen tissue section; lipid stains orange to red.

removes the vast majority of fat from sections, simply leaving an empty space within cells and tissues. Pathologists may be suspicious that these spaces previously contained fats, either in the form of lipid, lipoproteins or triglycerides, but they need to apply special stains such as oil red O and Sudan III to confirm its presence. For example, the presence of lipid within a poorly differentiated sarcoma may aid the further diagnosis of the tumour as a liposarcoma. Presence of lipid within vacuolated hepatocytes may aid diagnosis of a hepatic lipidosis, as opposed to a disease involving hepatic storage of other substances, such as glycogen. Figure 5.14 demonstrates the use of oil red O staining to highlight fat within vacuoles of neoplastic cells. This section is from one of multiple abdominal tumours in a horse which presented with marked and recurrent ascites. Oil red O stain on frozen sections together with immunohistochemical stains and electron microscopy confirmed the diagnosis of a lipid-rich mesothelioma in this case (Dobromylskyj et al. 2011).

Table 5.1 lists most (but not all) of the special stains and the features they look for.

Immunohistochemistry

Immunohistochemistry (IHC) is a molecular technique involving the localization of antigens in tissue sections by the use of a specific binding antibody. The interactions which occur between the antigen and antibody are then visualized by various methods, such as a fluorescent dye or an enzymatic colour change reaction. Such antigens, often referred to as 'markers', can be part of an infectious agent, foreign protein or a cell-surface receptor known to be present on specific cells or cell subsets.

IHC involves several steps, the number of which depends on the precise technique used, and whether it is a direct or indirect method. There is also sometimes an additional step to block non-specific background staining, using substances such as skimmed milk or normal serum. Background non-specific staining can occur for a number of reasons, including inadequate or delayed fixation of samples (for example in the centre of large tissue blocks), or endogenous enzyme activity or biotin within certain tissues.

In the direct method, a labelled antibody is used that directly detects the antigen within the tissues without the need for any further steps, making this technique short and simple to carry out. However, it is relatively insensitive compared to the indirect method, when an unlabelled primary antibody is then itself detected by labelled secondary antibody (directed against the species and isotype of the primary antibody). This results in amplification of the signal and thus increased sensitivity of the test. The secondary antibody can be labelled with a fluorescent dye (indirect immunofluorescence method) or with an enzyme such as peroxidase or alkaline phosphatase (indirect immunoenzyme method) which is then measured by the addition of a substrate to produce colorimetric end results.

Some other methods involve a third layer; for example, in the avidin-biotin complex (ABC) method the secondary antibody is conjugated to biotin, which then in turn forms a complex with avidin and peroxidase (Figure 5.15).

Positive and negative controls are always performed, to test the protocol is carried out correctly (positive control) and to check the specificity of any staining seen (negative control). An external positive control involves using tissue that is a known positive-staining sample, while an internal positive control consists of cells normally resident within the tissue that would be expected to stain positive (for example immunostaining of a skin biopsy for epithelial cell markers could use the epidermis as the internal positive control). Negative controls generally consist of omitting the primary antibody or replacing the

Table 5.1 Summary of the most commonly used special stains

	Abbreviation	Uses
Metachromatic		
Giemsa		Blood smears, fungi, mast cells, parasites
Toluidine blue		Mast cells, amyloid
Mallory's phosphotungstic acid haematoxylin	PTAH	All tissue components
Bacterial and fungal		
Gram/Twort		Gram +/–
Ziehl–Neelsen	ZN	Acid-fast bacteria, iron inclusion bodies
Periodic acid-Schiff	PAS	Fungi (living)
(+/– diastase digestion)		Glycogen
Grocott's methenamine silver stain	GMS	Fungi (dead and alive)
Warthin–Starry		Spirochetes
Wade–Fite		Leprosy bacilli
Amyloid/copper/calcium stains		
Congo red		Amyloid
Toluidine blue		Amyloid
Von Kossa		Calcium
Rhodanine		Copper
Rubeanic acid		Copper
Mucins		
Alcian blue		Acid mucins (proteoglycans)
Alcian blue/PAS		Acid and neutral mucins
Tissue components		
Masson's trichrome		Connective tissues
Gordon & Sweets		Reticulin, liver structure
Gomori hexamine silver		Basement membranes
Haematoxylin van Gieson	HVG	Collagen, muscle
Martius scarlet blue	MSB	Fibrin, connective tissue

Table 5.1 (continued)

	Abbreviation	Uses
Pigment stains		
Masson–Fontana		Melanin
Permanganate bleach		Removes melanin
Fouchet		Bile pigments
Perl's Prussian blue		Ferric iron
		Ferrous iron

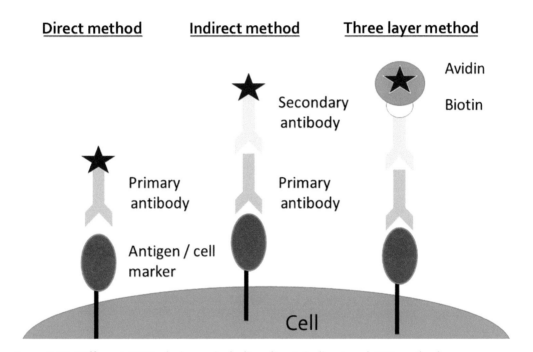

Figure 5.15 Different IHC techniques, including direct, indirect and ABC method.

primary antibody with an antibody that should not bind to any components of the tissue, in which case no positive staining should be present. This aids differentiation between non-specific and specific staining of cells.

There are several advantages to using IHC:

- the staining is highly specific to the target antigen
- the sensitivity is typically high due to amplification of the signal, since multiple antibodies can potentially bind to each antigen
- sensitivity can often be increased depending on the precise technique used

- the staining is visualized in situ which is important as it allows correlation of the antigen, be it a cell-surface marker or an infectious agent, with a specific cell population and/or lesion
- the technique uses routinely formalin-fixed tissues, so the same tissue sample can be used first for routine HE staining followed by IHC staining if required, without the need for further sampling of the patient.

Similar techniques can also be applied to suitable cytology preparations, a technique referred to as immunocytochemistry.

Infectious agents

Immunohistochemistry can be used to detect and confirm the presence of a particular infectious agent, for example, looking for feline coronavirus within macrophages in lesions suspicious for feline infectious peritonitis (FIP), which is currently the gold standard diagnostic test for this disease. Other infectious agents we can use IHC to detect include: feline calicivirus, feline herpesvirus 1, feline leukaemia virus, canine and feline parvovirus, canine distemper virus, *Toxoplasma gondii* and *Neospora caninum*. The technique has the advantages of detecting both viable and non-viable organisms, and is especially good for highlighting those present in only low numbers within suspicious-looking lesions.

There are several uses for IHC related to tumour diagnosis and prognostication, including differentiation of tumours, immunophenotyping of certain tumours such as lymphomas, assessment of proliferation markers such as Ki67 and of prognostic markers such as KIT staining patterns. All of these things can potentially have a great impact on the prognosis for a given case.

Tumour differentiation

The use of immunohistochemistry can often help guide the diagnosis of poorly differentiated neoplasms, but it is not always as straightforward as it might seem. Sometimes a stepwise approach is best, with the selection of which markers to use being dependent on the differential diagnoses and how distinction between different tumours will impact on clinical decision making, the treatment and prognosis for the patient. For some cases, more than one round of IHC staining might be most appropriate, to gain the maximum clinically useful information with minimal cost, but that would also increase the overall time taken to reach the diagnosis (or not). A definitive diagnosis may still not be guaranteed in these cases, but hopefully at least some differential diagnoses will be ruled in or out by any results obtained.

There are some basic rules to follow when deciding which IHC markers to use on a particular case, and when interpreting any ICH staining results.

- Always interpret IHC staining in conjunction with the HE slides.
- Positive and negative control slides are essential to interpretation.
- Try to avoid relying only on negative staining results.
- This often means using a panel of stains in varying combinations, not just single tests.
- Know your antibodies and how they behave.
- Do not expect neoplastic cells to follow the rules – they often do not!

Table 5.2 More commonly used IHC markers used in diagnosis of neoplasia

Target antigen	Cells stained	Uses
CD3	T-lymphocytes	Lymphoma
CD79a, CD20, Pax5	B-lymphocytes	Lymphoma
CD18, Iba-1, MHC class II	Histiocytes, leukocytes	Round cell tumours
Chromogranin A, Synaptophysin	Neuroendocrine cells	Neuroendocrine tumours
Cytokeratin (pan)	Epithelial cells	Carcinoma
c-KIT (CD117)	Haematopoietic stem cells	Mast cell tumours, GIST
Desmin	Muscle	Rhabdomyosarcoma
e-cadherin	Epithelial cells, Langerhans cells	Histiocytoma
GFAP	Glial cells	Tumours of glial origin
Glucagon, Insulin	Pancreatic hormones	Islet cell tumours
MelanA, PNL2	Melanocytes	Melanoma
MUM-1	Plasma cells	Plasma cell tumours
S100	Melanocytes, DCs, macrophages and more	Melanoma, others
Smooth muscle actin	Smooth muscle	Smooth muscle tumours
Vimentin	Mesenchymal cells	Sarcoma
Von Willebrands, CD31	Endothelial cells	Vascular tumours

Table 5.2 summarizes some of the more commonly used IHC markers used in diagnosis of neoplasia (not an exhaustive list). Each marker will have a specific staining pattern, depending on where that antigen is present in the target cell; this is important to know because it helps with interpretation, and to differentiate between real specific staining and non-specific background staining. Some markers will be cytoplasmic or membranous, others will be nuclear, some will vary.

As pathologists, we think of tumours as falling into one of three broad categories largely based on cell morphology and tumour growth pattern, namely epithelial (carcinoma if malignant), mesenchymal (sarcoma if malignant) and 'round cell' – although do note that technically round cell tumours are of mesenchymal cell origin. In cases of the most poorly differentiated neoplastic lesions, the pathologist often has few histological clues as to the origin of the tumour. At the most fundamental level, markers such as pancytokeratin and vimentin can aid identification of a mass as either a carcinoma or a sarcoma, respectively. Occasionally, tumours may express both markers (co-expression), for example as seen in mesotheliomas which can vary markedly in their histological appearance.

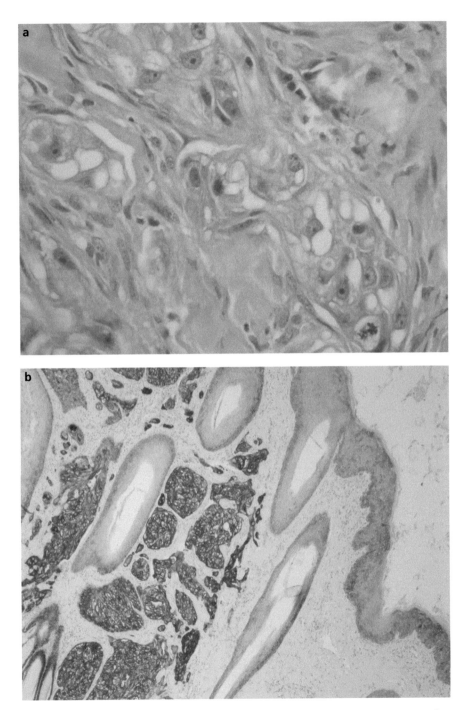

Figure 5.16 A poorly differentiated neoplasm in the skin of a dog with IHC staining for cytokeratin which is positive (brown). Note that the normal epithelium is also positive staining (epidermis and hair follicle epithelium, internal positive control).

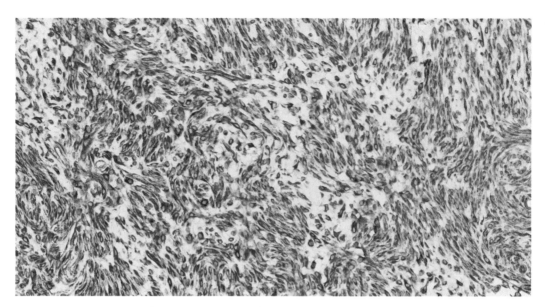

Figure 5.17 IHC staining for vimentin on a soft tissue tumour from a dog; spindle cell population is positive staining (brown).

Is it a carcinoma or a sarcoma?

If neoplastic cells are pancytokeratin positive and vimentin negative that typically indicates an epithelial neoplasm and, if malignant, then carcinoma (Figure 5.16). If neoplastic cells are pancytokeratin negative and vimentin positive that normally indicates a mesenchymal cell neoplasm and, if malignant, then sarcoma (Figure 5.17). If neoplastic cells are pancytokeratin positive and vimentin positive, there are a very small number of instances when this may occur, one of which includes a mesothelioma (Figure 5.18).

It is a carcinoma, but what type?

There are some more specific markers for epithelial neoplasms, but not perhaps as many as there are for sarcomas and round cell tumours. Those we will sometimes use include the neuroendocrine markers (chromogranin A and synaptophysin, Figure 5.19), hormone markers (insulin, glucagon for Islet cell tumours) and markers for thyroid origin (thyroglobulin, thyroid transcription factor 1 (TTF1), not entirely specific for thyroid as some lung tumours also express), uroplakin III and WT-1 (urothelial carcinoma) together with more specific types of cytokeratin, which can add further information.

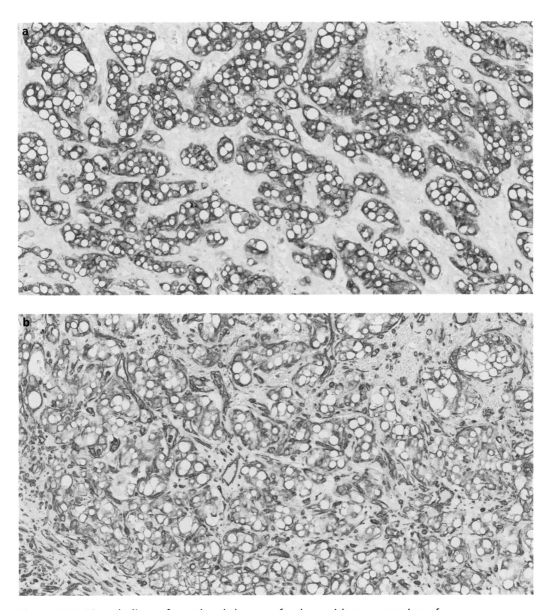

Figure 5.18 Mesothelioma from the abdomen of a dog, with co-expression of
(a) cytokeratin and (b) vimentin. Some other poorly differentiated tumours may also do
this on occasion.

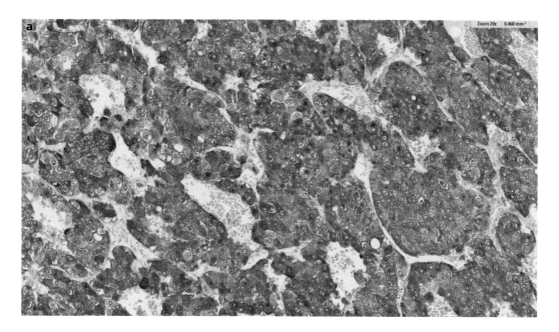

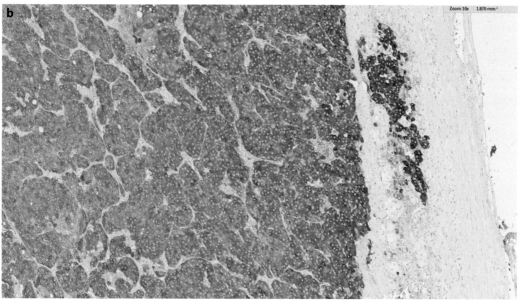

Figure 5.19 A canine adrenal mass with IHC staining for (a) chromogranin A and (b) synaptophysin are both positive, consistent with a phaeochromocytoma in this case.

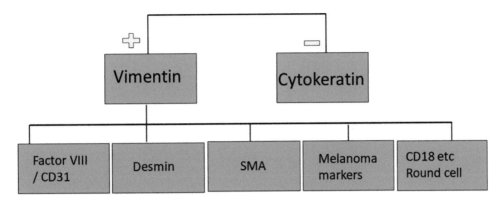

Figure 5.20 **If a tumour is a sarcoma, what further markers are available to differentiate it further?**

It is a sarcoma, but what type?

For tumours with a spindle cell morphology, and which are vimentin positive, there is a set of more specific markers which may then be considered, depending on the differential diagnosis list. Since some (amelanotic) melanomas and round cell tumours (histiocytic sarcoma) can also be spindle-shaped they may or may not also be on the differential list (Figure 5.20). These include:

haemangiosarcoma:	CD31, von Willebrands factor (factor VIII)
muscle origin (e.g. rhabdomyosarcoma):	Desmin
smooth muscle origin (leiomyosarcoma):	smooth muscle actin (SMA)
gastrointestinal stromal tumour (GIST):	c-KIT
liposarcoma:	S100
histiocytic sarcoma:	CD18, MHC class II, Iba-1
melanoma:	S100, PNL2, MelanA

It looks like a round cell tumour, but what type?

For tumours with a round cell morphology, there is a longer list of markers and differentials, including those below. Amelanotic melanomas could also make an appearance here as well (Figure 5.21).

lymphoma:	CD3 (T-cell), CD79a/CD20/Pax5 (B-cell +/−plasma cell)
plasma cell tumour:	MUM-1 (also mature B-cells), kappa/lambda
mast cell tumour:	c-KIT, mast cell tryptase, (Giemsa/Toluidine blue)
histiocytic origin, with varying degrees of specificity:	CD18, MHC class II, Iba-1, e-cadherin, CD204 (histiocytoma, histiocytic sarcoma, histiocytosis)
melanoma again:	S100, PNL2, MelanA

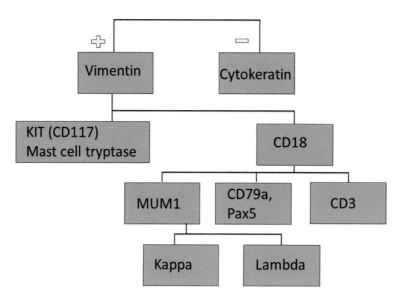

Figure 5.21 An IHC panel for a tumour with a round cell morphology may look like this.

Kappa and lambda are two types of light chain that exist as part of an antibody. Each individual plasma cell can only produce one type of light chain, either kappa or lambda. Therefore, a normal (inflammatory, non-neoplastic) population of plasma cells will contain a mixture of cells each producing either kappa or lambda light chain (Figure 5.22). Whereas a neoplastic plasma cell population (derived from a single malignant cell or clone) will produce light chain of only one type, either kappa or lambda but not a mixture of both (Figure 5.23). So, not only can these be used as IHC markers for plasma cell tumours, but they can also differentiate between a neoplastic cell population and an inflammatory one.

Tumour prognostication using IHC

Immunophenotyping of lymphomas

Lymphomas can generally be immunophenotyped as of B-lymphocyte origin (CD79a/Pax5/CD20 positive) or T-lymphocyte origin (CD3 positive). Occasionally we see null-cell lymphomas (also known as non-B-/non-T-cell) which are CD3, Pax5 and CD79a negative. This is a very uncommon variant reported to constitute 0.8–2% of canine lymphomas, potentially thought to arise from a third subset of lymphocytes called natural killer cells. Also, occasionally we see lymphomas that demonstrate dual positivity; apparent co-expression of both B-cell and T-cell markers is unusual in a lymphoma, but this pattern can be seen in a small proportion of T-cell lymphomas (most authors call these T-cell lymphomas, but the lineage is not universally accepted). About 10% of human T-cell tumours may show this immunostaining pattern. In dogs, this pattern is associated with antigen receptor rearrangement and with loss of chromosomes, both strong markers of malignancy. There may also be an increased risk of leukaemia for lymphoid tumours with this expression pattern.

Immunophenotyping is essential for World Health Organization (WHO) classification of lymphomas, which cannot be applied without knowing whether a lymphoma is of B-cell or T-cell origin.

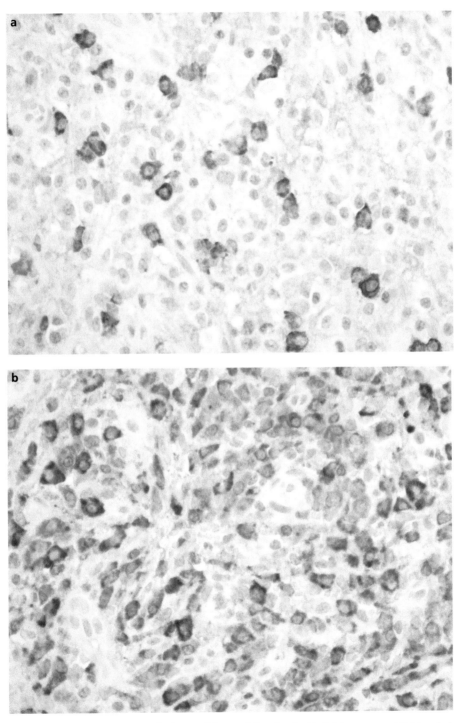

Figure 5.22 Feline plasma cell pododermatitis, positive for both (a) kappa and (b) lambda, consistent with an inflammatory cell population of plasma cells.

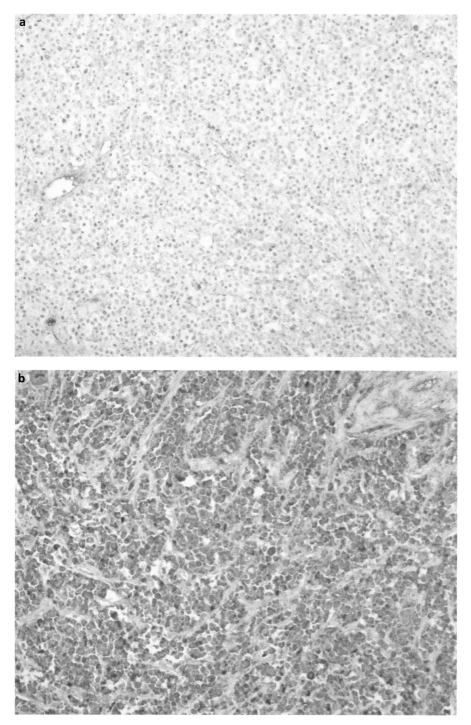

Figure 5.23 Canine plasma cell tumour, with negative staining for (a) kappa and (b) positive staining for lambda, consistent with a neoplastic process of plasma cell origin.

Immunophenotyping and classification of canine lymphoma is an important prognostic tool and may also help guide therapeutic decision making. Below is an example of WHO classification of a canine lymphoma (Figure 5.24).

Case study (Figure 5.24)

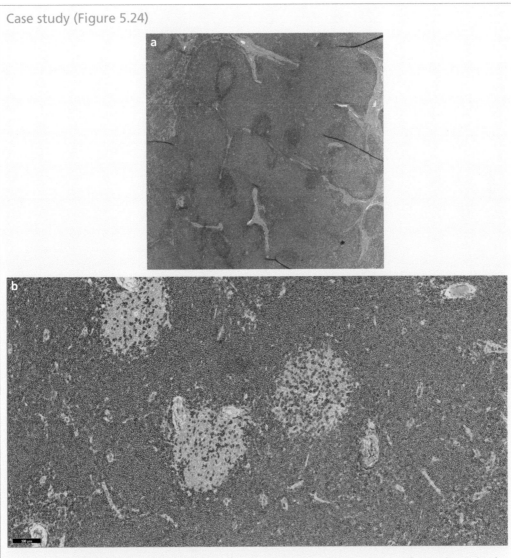

Figure 5.24 (a) HE section at low-power of canine lymph node. Expansion of a medium-sized lymphoid population, minimal atypia and very low mitotic rate. There is displacement of somewhat fading lymphoid follicles, and an increased amount of fibrous stroma present, supportive of an underlying TZL, but IHC is required to confirm. (b) CD3-immunostaining of the lymph node shows the expanded lymphoid population is of T-cell origin (brown cytoplasmic staining). Remaining follicles are negative staining, leaving blue spaces in a sea of brown. (c) CD79a immunostaining shows the normal residual B-cells in fading follicles (brown cytoplasmic). (d) Pax 5 immunostaining shows similar features (B-cells, nuclear stain, brown).

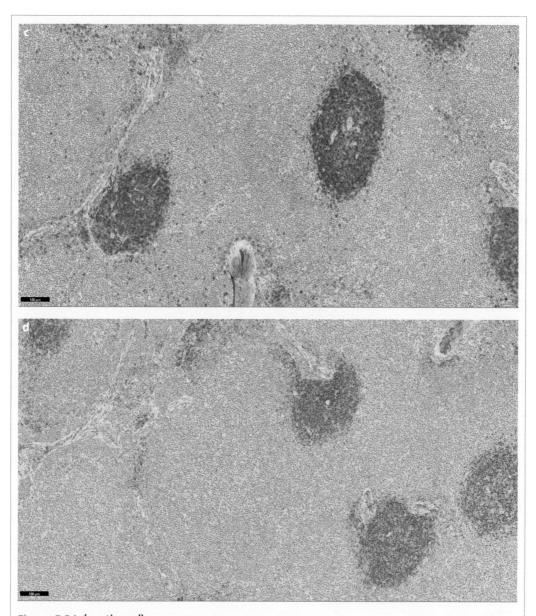

Figure 5.24 (continued)

A clinically well, middle-aged, crossbreed dog presenting with enlargement of only the submandibular lymph nodes. Cytology revealed an expanded population of medium-sized lymphoid cells of
uncertain significance, with atypical hyperplasia or indolent lymphoma as potential differential diagnoses. Wedge biopsy submitted for histological assessment confirmed expansion of a medium-sized
lymphoid population and also marked distortion of the normal lymph node architecture; there was
minimal atypia and the mitotic rate was very low. IHC staining confirmed the expanded lymphoid

population was composed of T-cells (CD3 positive) while IHC staining for B-cells showed how the fading lymphoid follicles were being displaced. The morphology of the cells, the distortion of the lymph node architecture and the IHC staining pattern taken all together were consistent with a T-zone lymphoma (TZL). TZL is a peripheral T-cell lymphoma of small cell type, which has a tendency to remain localized for long periods and is characterized by little impairment of general health and often long survival with minimal therapy. The typical presentation is usually enlargement of one or two nodes, often found incidentally.

Assessment of KIT patterns in canine mast cell tumours

KIT is a tyrosine kinase receptor normally present on the cell surface (that is, membrane-associated), and changes in KIT staining patterns in tumour cells is used in canine mast cell tumour (MCT) prognostication (Figure 5.25). Normal mast cells demonstrate membrane-associated staining only (staining pattern I) and this pattern is retained in some MCTs. In some other MCTs, however, a proportion of neoplastic cells show intense focal or stippled cytoplasmic staining (pattern II) or diffuse cytoplasmic staining (pattern III). Staining patterns II and III, that is, increased cytoplasmic staining of KIT, are thought to be associated with shorter overall survival times and increased risk of local recurrence (there is some disagreement about the significance of pattern II between different groups).

Proliferation markers (Ki67 and MCM7)

Ki67 is a nuclear protein expressed in all active phases of the cell cycle but which is not present in non-cycling cells. The relative number of Ki67 positive cells indicates the *growth fraction* within a tumour cell population. The most well-known example of diagnostic use of Ki67 is in canine MCT prognostication, where studies have suggested that it is possible to divide intermediate-grade (Patnaik grade II) tumours into two groups based on the Ki67 score (Figure 5.26). There is also on-going research into the potential use of the Ki67 index in other tumours such as canine oral melanoma.

MCM7 is another proliferation marker that has also been studied in canine MCTs. Similar to Ki67, it is possible to divide intermediate-grade (Patnaik grade II) tumours into two groups based on the MCM7 score (Figure 5.27).

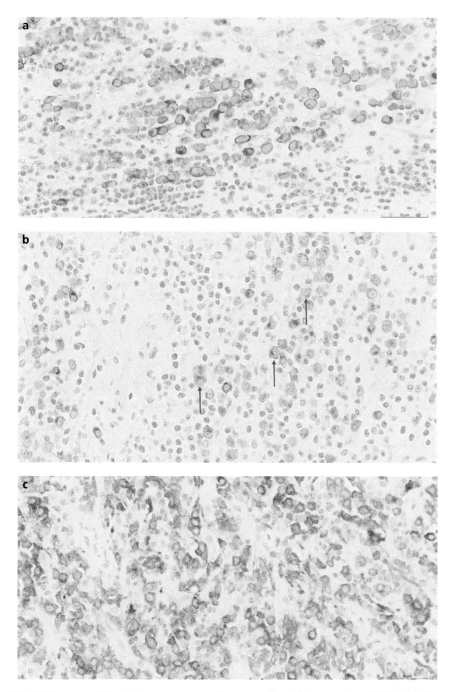

Figure 5.25 Different c-KIT staining patterns of mast cells within a canine MCT: (a) KIT staining pattern I, membrane-associated staining only; (b) KIT staining pattern II, loss of membrane-associated staining with focal or stippled cytoplasmic staining (red arrows); (c) KIT staining pattern III, diffuse cytoplasmic staining.

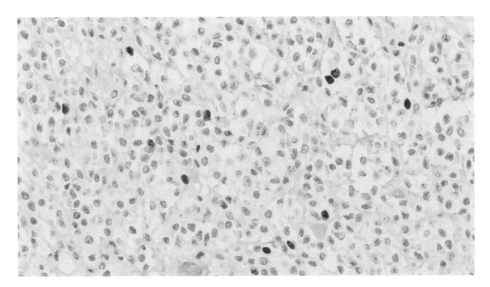

Figure 5.26 Ki67 immunostaining of a canine MCT: positive (brown) nuclear staining of some of the neoplastic cells.

100 μm

Figure 5.27 MCM7 immunostaining of a feline MCT: positive (brown) nuclear staining of neoplastic mast cells (sadly, not shown to be a useful prognostic marker for feline MCTs) (Dobromylskyj et al., 2015).

PARR and other PCR-based tests

How PCR works

In basic terms, PCR detects a region of interest within DNA, by the use of a pair of sequence-specific primers. Primers are a short segment of base pairs, designed to match small but highly specific areas of the genetic code ('area of interest'). Under correct conditions, primers will bind to that area of interest and nowhere else. Primer design is thus key to an accurate, specific and reliable PCR test.

Double-stranded DNA is first denatured into two separate strands by heating to 95°C. Primer pairs then bind to specific sites on each of the two strands (which is why primers always come in pairs), a process which is temperature-specific depending on any given pair of primers (typically in the range of 50–60°C). Once the primers are annealed, the sample is heated to 72°C, at which temperature the enzyme DNA-polymerase is active and extends the primer sequence using the DNA strand as a template, thus producing copies of each of the original DNA strands. Each cycle theoretically doubles the number of copies of that particular area of the DNA in the sample. This thermal cycling is repeated many times until the amplified DNA fragment is present at detectable levels (Figure 5.28). Different forms of PCR use different techniques for detection – traditional PCR uses electrophoresis to separate out different lengths of DNA fragments according to size, within an agarose gel. Ethidium bromide is added to the buffer; it binds to DNA molecules in the gel and when the gel is illuminated by UV light, it allows bands of DNA in the gel to be visualized (Figure 5.29). Quantitative PCR involves fluorescent probes for both detection and more accurate measurement of the number of DNA fragments (actually the measurement is of the number of cycles required to hit a certain threshold or number of DNA fragments, normally referred to as the Ct value).

Therefore, PCR has many uses: for genotyping; looking at gene expression (via messenger RNA); detection of DNA/RNA of infectious agents; looking for genetic mutations (such as in the c-KIT gene as part of MCT prognostication) and also as part of PARR testing.

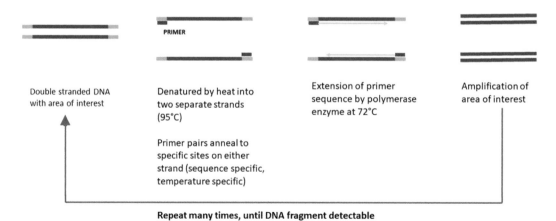

Double stranded DNA with area of interest

Denatured by heat into two separate strands (95°C)

PRIMER

Primer pairs anneal to specific sites on either strand (sequence specific, temperature specific)

Extension of primer sequence by polymerase enzyme at 72°C

Amplification of area of interest

Repeat many times, until DNA fragment detectable

Figure 5.28 Schematic representation of how a PCR cycle works.

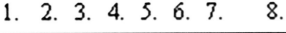

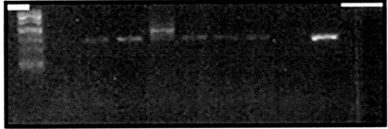

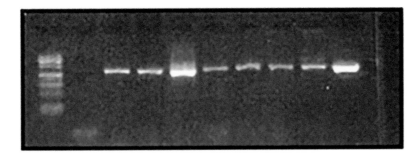

Figure 5.29 **PCR products on an agarose gel, viewed under UV light.**

PARR testing

PARR testing is a PCR-based assay; it stands for 'PCR for Antigen Receptor Rearrangements'. To understand how PARR works, we first have to revisit how T-cell receptor genes and immunoglobulin heavy chains work normally to provide such a large variety of T-cell and B-cell clones in the immune system. In the germline, these receptors have multiple genes, with multiple versions of each gene present. As part of lymphocyte development and maturation, these will rearrange, so that each clone has a different 'set' of genes as part of their T-cell or B-cell (immunoglobulin heavy chain) receptor. For simplification, let us focus on the V-gene. Let us say each clone rearranges so that it contains a single V-gene that is then encoding for part of that particular clone's receptor. In an inflammatory process, multiple lymphocyte clones are expanded in number; each clone has a different length of DNA encoding its TCR (or B-cell equivalent) due to this process of gene rearrangement. The PCR primers therefore pick up DNA fragments which are different in length to each other, giving a polyclonal pattern (Figure 5.30).

In a neoplastic process, only a single lymphocyte clone is expanded to form the cell population present. All (or very nearly all) of the lymphocytes in that tissue will have the same gene rearrangement, and the PCR primers will therefore only amplify that one version, and all of the DNA products will be of the same length. This gives a single peak on the graph, that is, monoclonal (Figure 5.31).

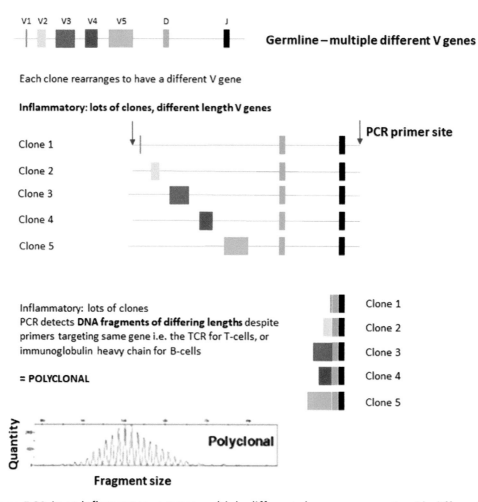

Figure 5.30 In an inflammatory process multiple different clones are present, with different size fragments detected and amplified by the PCR reaction, giving multiple peaks.

Points to note

Like any test, PARR has its limitations, and it is important to be aware of these, both when considering requesting the test and also when interpreting the results. It is important to remember that the PARR does not necessarily indicate the immunophenotype of any lymphoma (due to more rearrangement of genes, T-cell lymphomas can occasionally show clonality of the BCR and vice versa!). Therefore, IHC (or other tests such as flow cytology) is still needed for immunophenotyping, in conjunction with the original histological findings for WHO classification. It may seem tempting to skip IHC and go straight for PARR testing, but this is not advisable, as it is important that the findings of each of these tests are considered together. Partly this is because both false negatives and false positive results do occur with PARR, just as with any test.

False negatives and false positives can both arise because of relatively poor sequence coverage of the TCR and BCR regions on which the design of the PCR primers used for PARR testing is based

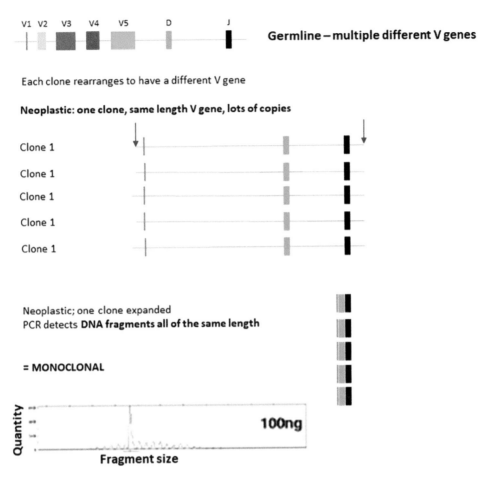

Figure 5.31 In a neoplastic process, a single clone is present, and so only a fragment of one length is detected and amplified by the PCR reaction, giving a single peak.

(especially in cats – due to a relative lack of sequencing data across populations). So, it is possible that not all clones are detected by the primers used in any given test. False negative results may also occur if the sample does not contain sufficient neoplastic cells or if the DNA is of poor quality, then very little may be detected at all. False positives can potentially arise when there is detection of a low number of clones (oligoclonal) when interpretation can be challenging. This could possibly be due to immune-mediated diseases, or infectious diseases which result in clonal expansion of only one or very few clones, as opposed to a broader selection of clones as seen in the more typical inflammatory response.

ISH/FISH

In situ hybridization (ISH) and one of its subtypes fluorescence in situ hybridization (FISH) are molecular techniques that use a labelled complementary probe to bind to and localize a specific sequence of DNA or RNA within a tissue sample. When the probe is labelled with a fluorescent marker and viewed with a fluorescent microscope the probe can be visualized on the slide.

Similar to IHC, there are several advantages to using ISH:

- the staining is highly specific to the target DNA/RNA sequence
- the staining is visualized in situ, which allows correlation of the DNA/RNA with specific tissues and/or lesion
- the technique uses routinely formalin-fixed tissues, so the same tissue sample can be used first for routine HE staining followed by ISH staining if required, without the need for further sampling of the patient.

Depending on the target, ISH can be used to look for particular genetic code in individual cells, such as specific genes or parts of genes, and then map them to particular chromosomes for example – this might be done looking for chromosomal abnormalities.

Another widespread use of FISH is the identification of pathogens in tissues, for example, in gastrointestinal biopsies to look for eubacteria located within the tissues. When there is also evidence of clustering this suggests the microbes have been multiplying in the tissues themselves (as opposed to being present within the luminal contents and/or implanted during sampling). An initial screen may use a non-specific probe which will detect nucleic acid from any eubacteria. If found, more specific probes can be used to further identify the bacteria as *E. coli*, *Salmonella*, *Campylobacter* and so on.

There has been recent interest in the use of FISH to study bacteria present in a range of conditions in cats and dogs, including gall bladder mucocoeles, enterocolitis, intestinal lymphoma, endocarditis and inflammatory liver disease, among others.

Self-assessment: 'What's your diagnosis?'

Case 1

A 9-year 6-month-old female (neutered) domestic short hair cat presents with an intestinal mass, which is surgically resected and submitted for histopathology.

Figure 5.32c shows the results of the immunohistochemical stains for T-lymphocytes and B-lymphocytes. What immunophenotype do you think this lymphoma is, T-cell or B-cell?

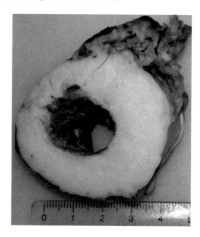

Figure 5.32a Appearance on gross assessment of the formalin-fixed specimen. The full circumference of the intestine is expanded by a soft, homogenous cream mass, with loss of the normal layering.

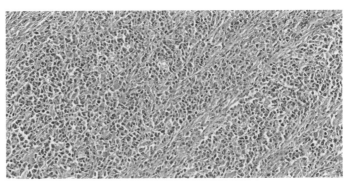

Figure 5.32b Histological appearance, at high power, stained with HE. The diagnosis is of an intestinal lymphoma, diffuse, large cell, with a high mitotic count. Immunohistochemical staining is performed.

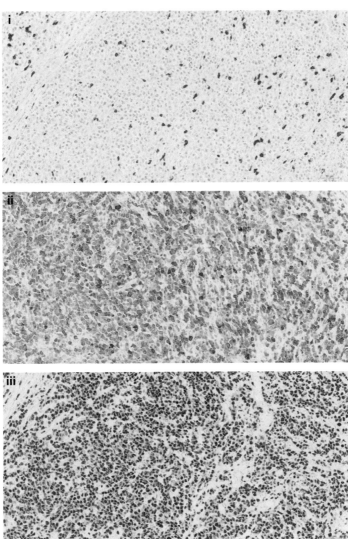

Figure 5.32c (i) CD3 stain; (ii) CD79a stain; (iii) Pax5 stain.

Case 2

A 4-year-old male (neutered) domestic long hair cat has had a submandibular swelling for 2 months. He has access to outdoors, is fully vaccinated and a known hunter of small rodents. He is systemically well and has no other lesions on physical examination. The swelling has not responded to a 2 week course of broad spectrum antibiotic medication. A biopsy is taken for histopathological assessment (Figure 5.33a).

1. Based on this initial assessment, what are your differential diagnoses?
2. What additional special stains might you request and why?
3. Looking at Figure 5.33b, can you identify this special stain, and is it positive or negative in this case?

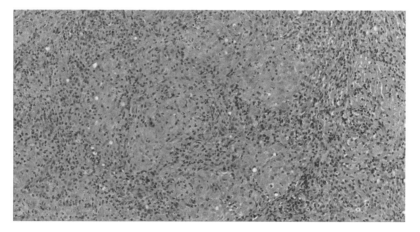

Figure 5.33a Histological appearance, at high power, stained with HE. There is a marked, diffuse and locally extensive, mixed inflammatory cell infiltrate present, which includes clusters and aggregates of reactive macrophages together with variable numbers of neutrophils, some lymphocytes and plasma cells.

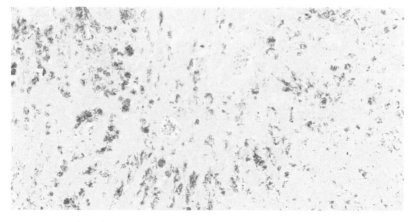

Figure 5.33b Can you identify this special stain, and is it positive or negative in this case?

Case 3

A 10-year-old male (neutered) Maine coon cat presents to your clinic with a history of acute collapse, which is found to be due to a haemoabdomen. On exploratory laparotomy, a ruptured splenic mass is discovered and a splenectomy performed. Representative sections are submitted for histopathology (Figure 5.34a).

1. What types of sarcoma can arise in the spleen of both dogs and cats, and which is of most concern in this case?
2. What immunohistochemical stains might be suggested in this case?
3. Immunohistochemical staining is performed (Figure 5.34b) with the following:
    a vimentin – is the neoplastic cell population positive or negative staining? What does this tell us?
    b CD31 and factor VIII (von Willebrand's factor) – is the neoplastic cell population positive or negative staining? What does this tell us?
4. What is your final diagnosis in this case?

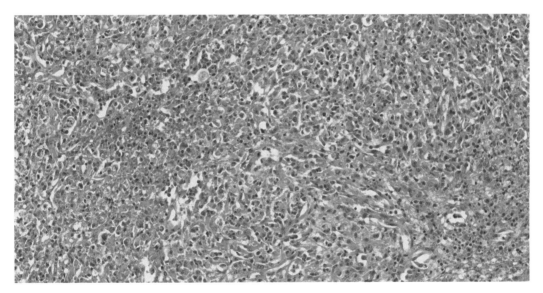

Figure 5.34a HE stained section showing parts of an unencapsulated, infiltrative neoplastic mass associated with extensive areas of necrosis and haemorrhage. The appearance is most consistent with a sarcoma. In some fields, there appears to be formation of vascular spaces lined by the neoplastic cells, but elsewhere the growth pattern is more solid.

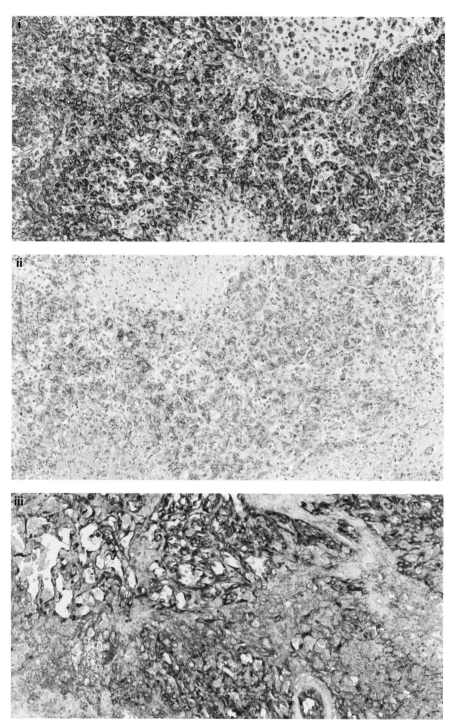

Figure 5.34b Immunohistochemical staining: (i) vimentin ; (ii) CD31; (iii) factor VIII (von Willebrand's factor).

Case 4

A 5-month-old male domestic long hair kitten presents with an area of scabbing and crusting under the left nostril (Figure 5.35a), but no obvious nasal or ocular discharge, no other lesions on the skin or evidence of fleas. The owner reports that a sibling has a similar facial lesion.

1. Skin biopsies are submitted for histopathology. What might your list of possible differential diagnoses include at this stage?

Figure 5.35b shows a HE stained section at lower power, through haired skin and the keratin layer. It shows hyperplasia of the epidermis (acanthosis) and also hyperkeratosis. There is a mild, perivascular to interstitial, mixed dermatitis.

2. Can you identify the objects within the keratin layer, highlighted by the red arrows?

Figure 5.35c shows a higher power view of the HE stained section.

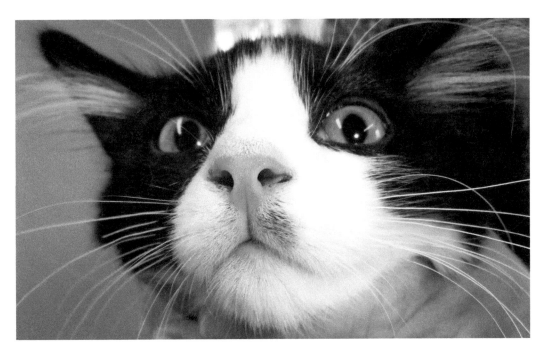

Figure 5.35a Photograph of the lesion.

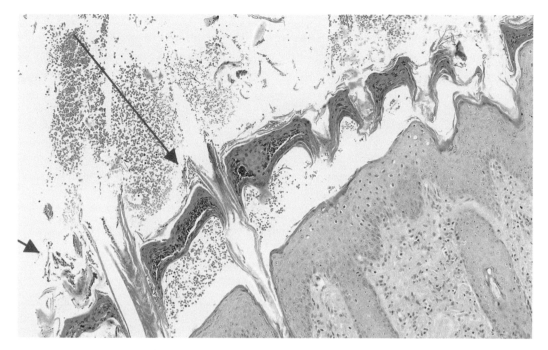

Figure 5.35b A HE stained section at lower power.

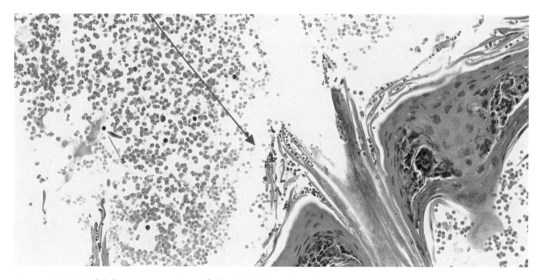

Figure 5.35c A higher power view of the HE stained section.

3. What special stains which you suggest in this case?
4. Can you identify this stain in Figure 5.35d?

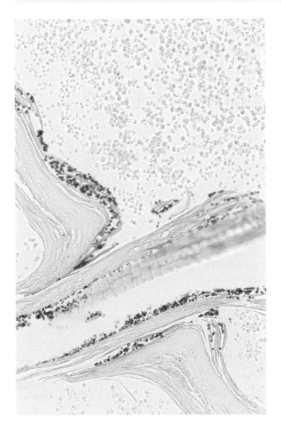

Figure 5.35d **Can you identify this stain?**

The answers are available on page 176.

6

Oncology: recognizing features of neoplasia and of malignancy

Introduction

In this chapter, we will take a look at some of the features of neoplasia and also of malignancy. This chapter is illustrated throughout by a large number of real cases, including comparing benign and malignant tumours arising from the same cell type, looking at some of the hallmarks of differentiation and also at why differentiating between inflammatory and neoplastic lesions can sometimes be extremely challenging.

Nomenclature

Before we start, it is best to consider some nomenclature and basic definitions. The word neoplasm literally means 'new growth', and this can be in reference to either benign or malignant processes. The word tumour translates as 'swelling' – as in the five cardinal signs of inflammation being tumour (swelling), rubor (redness), calor (heat), dolor (pain) and loss of function (functio laesa). Tumours can also be considered either benign or malignant. The word cancer (meaning 'crab') is typically only used to denote a malignant process.

To the pathologist, a benign tumour is one which does not invade the surrounding tissue or spread to new anatomic locations within the body. Malignant tumours, if left untreated, will invade locally, may spread by metastasis (meaning 'change of place') and will ultimately kill the host.

It is important to remember that tumour development is a stepwise process and there are a number of potentially pre-neoplastic changes which may in themselves be significant (Figure 6.1).

- *Hyperplasia* – an increased cell number within a tissue. For example, epidermal hyperplasia is seen as a part of normal wound repair.
- *Hypertrophy* (not to be confused with *hyperplasia*) – an increase in cell size not cell number. For example, by skeletal muscle in response to workload.
- *Metaplasia* – the transformation of one differentiated cell type into another type.
- *Dysplasia* – an abnormal pattern of tissue growth, for example, a disorderly arrangement of cells within epithelium

Pre-neoplastic changes

Pre-neoplastic changes can indicate an increased risk of neoplasia developing and may themselves progress to neoplasia. They also tend to be reversible changes. Dysplasia and metaplasia are terms that can also be applied to tumours to describe changes that persist during the transition from pre-neoplasia to neoplasia, that is, there may be areas of dysplasia and metaplasia present within or associated with a neoplasm. Hyperplasia and hypertrophy are not appropriate in descriptions of true neoplasms although they may be present in surrounding tissues. Dysplasia can also occur for other reasons, such as a result of chronic inflammation or injury, and we will consider this later when talking about the challenges of distinguishing between some inflammatory and neoplastic processes.

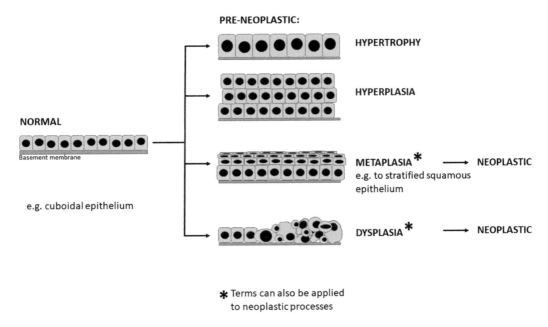

Figure 6.1 Differences between hypertrophy, hyperplasia, metaplasia and dysplasia.

Table 6.1 Characteristics of benign versus malignant tumours

Characteristic	Benign tumour	Malignant tumour
Differentiation	Well-differentiated appearance Structure similar to tissue of origin Little or no anaplasia	Usually, some lack of differentiation Structure often atypical Variable degree of anaplasia
Growth rate	Slow Progressive expansion Rare mitotic figures Normal appearing mitotic figures	Slow to rapid growth Erratic growth rate Mitotic figures increased Mitotic figures can be abnormal
Local Invasion	No invasion Cohesive and expansile growth Capsule often present	Local invasion Infiltrative growth Often no capsule
Metastasis	No metastasis	Frequent metastasis (the definitive criterion for malignancy)

Benign versus malignant tumours

Table 6.1 summarizes the characteristics of benign versus malignant tumours, although this is rather a sweeping generalization; each type of tumour is somewhat unique, and this is where the experience and knowledge of a pathologist comes into play as part of interpretation. For example, the level at which the mitotic rate would be considered as 'increased' for a particular type of tumour is partly dependent on what the normal (baseline) mitotic rate would be for that particular population. As an illustration of this, basal epithelial cells divide as part of their normal function, and so a benign tumour of basal cell origin would demonstrate a degree of mitotic activity that in another cell type might be alarming but in a basal cell tumour merely reflects the normal cell behaviour.

There follows some examples of benign tumours with their malignant counterparts, to illustrate some of the differences we see as pathologists.

Lipoma versus liposarcoma

Figure 6.2a shows a lipoma from a dog, a benign neoplasm arising from adipocytes. The tumour cells closely resemble their non-neoplastic counterparts. It can be impossible to distinguish the well-differentiated fat cells present in a lipoma from those seen in normal adipose tissue, unless the overall growth pattern can be seen. These tumours are typically well-circumscribed, non-encapsulated, soft and white to yellow. The majority are slow-growing expansile masses and are cured by excision, although some have a history of more rapid growth, and we also see infiltrative forms which can be more challenging to completely excise.

Figure 6.2b shows a liposarcoma (presumptive) also from a dog, the malignant counterpart of a lipoma. Note that only some of the neoplastic cells contain the characteristic circular, clear and sharply delineated cytoplasmic vacuole, and that where present the vacuole varies considerably in size. There is also variation in cell and nuclear size, with nuclear atypia (more on this later). This tissue no longer resembles mature adipose tissue.

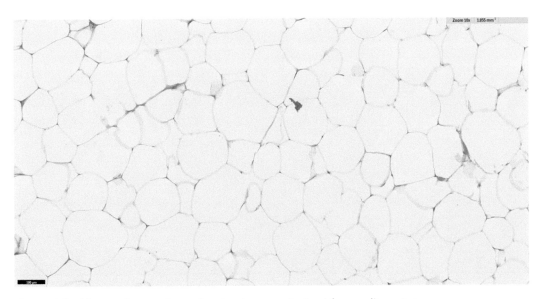

Figure 6.2a Lipoma from a dog, a benign tumour derived from adipocytes.

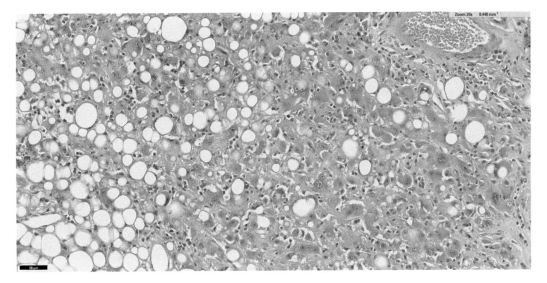

Figure 6.2b Liposarcoma from a dog, the malignant counterpart of a lipoma.

Haemangioma versus haemangiosarcoma

The two images in Figure 6.3a are from a cutaneous haemangioma from a dog. The low-power view shows this mass is well-demarcated and expansile in nature. The high-power view shows blood-filled spaces lined by a single cell layer; the neoplastic cells resemble normal endothelial cells, there is no cellular or nuclear atypia, and no mitotic activity.

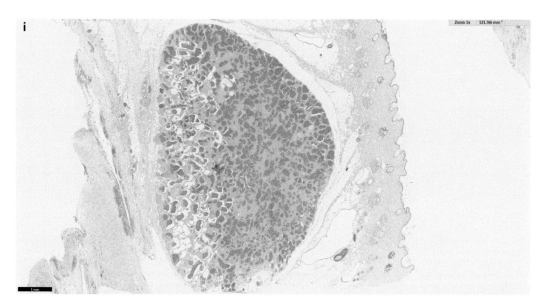

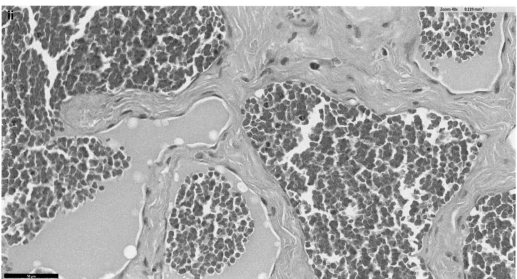

Figure 6.3a Cutaneous haemangioma from a dog, a benign neoplasm arising from endothelial cells.

Figure 6.3b shows a splenic haemangiosarcoma from a dog. The tumour cells no longer closely resemble endothelial cells; they vary in size and shape, and form somewhat irregular channels and spaces. There is mitotic activity, with nuclear pleomorphism and prominent nucleoli.

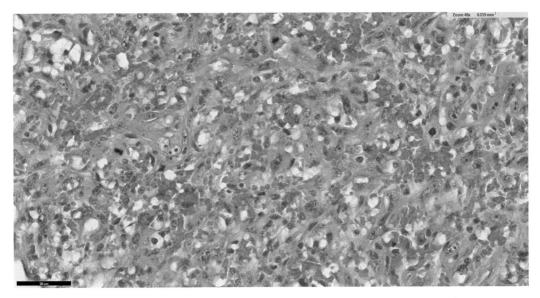

Figure 6.3b Splenic haemangiosarcoma from a dog, the malignant counterpart of haemangioma.

Hepatoma versus hepatocellular carcinoma

Figure 6.4a shows a benign hepatocellular tumour or 'hepatoma'. The neoplastic cells closely resemble hepatocytes although with some variation in cell and nuclear size. The key diagnostic feature is the loss of tissue architecture; the cells no longer form cords lining sinusoids, and portal tracts are absent. The mass has an expansile growth pattern and compresses the surrounding liver parenchyma, from which it is well-demarcated.

Figure 6.4b shows a mass in the pancreas of a dog. The tumour cells are poorly differentiated, and it took me a while to figure out this was of hepatocellular origin. The mass was largely necrotic and poorly demarcated. In a few fields, the cells still vaguely resemble hepatocytes but with marked vacuolation, nuclear and cellular atypia and mitotic activity (red arrow). There is no normal architecture, but there was apparent lymphovascular invasion. I called this a carcinoma, probably hepatocellular in origin, poorly differentiated.

Hallmarks of differentiation

Hallmarks of differentiation are features we can look for when trying to determine whether something is neoplastic or otherwise. This can take the form of morphological changes, or changes in function, and can occur at different levels – tissue, cell or nucleus.

At the tissue level, we can look for loss of the normal features of cellular morphology and organization, which is often associated with loss of functional capacity. This may be reflected in a *loss of normal tissue architecture*, for example, in a lymph node where the normal tissue architecture is lost with the development of lymphoma (see Chapter 3). This may also take the form of *loss of an orderly pattern of maturation* of cells. An example would be the loss of the normal pattern of epidermal maturation seen with squamous cell carcinoma (SCC), resulting in features such as keratin pearl formation and invasion

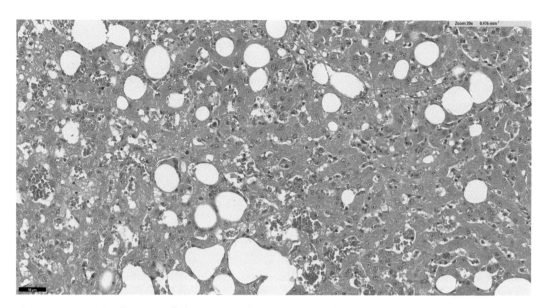

Figure 6.4a Benign hepatocellular tumour from the liver of a dog.

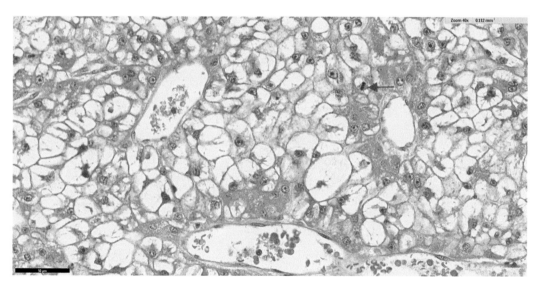

Figure 6.4b Malignant neoplasm, located within the pancreas of a dog and presumed to be metastatic from a primary liver tumour; presumed hepatocellular origin. Red arrow highlights a mitotic figure.

of epithelial cells through the basement membrane. The changes seen in the epidermis are really a good illustration of what we see in normal, hyperplastic, dysplastic and finally neoplastic processes (Figure 6.5). You will see changes in the architecture, loss of normal pattern of maturation, changes to cellular and nuclear morphology and also to the growth pattern.

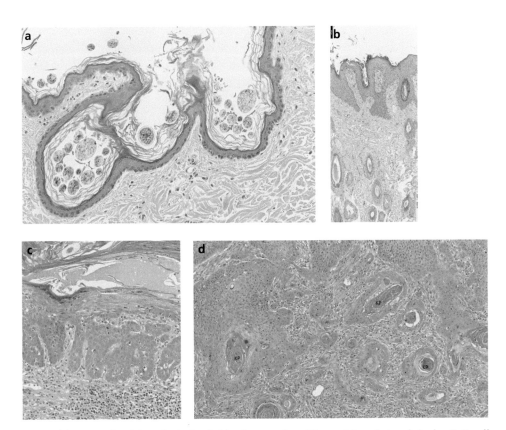

Figure 6.5 (a) Normal epidermis, haired skin from a dog. The epidermis tends to be 3–5 cells thick, with a normal and orderly maturation from the basement membrane lined by the basal layer (stratum basale) through the stratum spinosum, stratum granulosum and stratum lucidum to the stratum corneum, covered superficially by a layer of keratin. (b) Hyperplastic epidermis, from a dog with chronic dermatitis. There is an increased number of cells, with some of the layers expanded, but overall, the pattern of maturation is maintained. The basal layer has an undulating appearance, with formation of rete pegs, but the basement membrane is intact and there is no invasive growth. There may be mitotic activity, but it is confined to the basal layer (appropriately). (c) Dysplastic epidermis or 'carcinoma in situ' – an example from the haired skin of a cat's pinna, with actinic keratosis (AK), also known as actinic carcinoma in situ, or solar keratosis. There is loss of orderly maturation and architectural distortion resulting from loss of polarity of some keratinocytes within the basal and spinous layers. There is mild nuclear atypia, with some nuclear enlargement, nucleolar prominence and occasional mitotic figures noted above the basal layer (abnormal). Occasional scattered apoptotic cells are also present, but there is no breaching of the basement membrane or invasive growth. This is considered the prodromal phase in the development of UV light related SCC. (d) Neoplastic epidermis – this is a case of SCC arising from the pinna of a cat. Note the frequent nests and small islands of epithelial cells present in the dermis, with no apparent connection to the overlying epidermis. This implies invasive growth with breaching of the basement membrane. There is loss of orderly maturation, and epithelial cells demonstrate marked nuclear atypia, increased mitotic activity and there is formation of keratin pearls (indicated by 'KP') – where squamous differentiation and keratinization occurs within the small nests and islands, rather than at the surface of the epidermis where it should occur.

Alternatively, this change may take the form of either a *loss or gain of function*. For example, neoplastic cells arising from alveolar lining cells of the lung are generally unable to perform normal respiratory function. Some tumours retain normal function, but their functionality is no longer regulated as it should be, such as thyroid adenomas causing hyperthyroidism in cats (Figure 6.6), or plasma cell tumours causing hypergammaglobulinaemia.

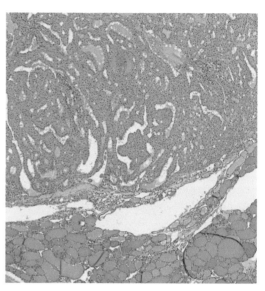

Figure 6.6a Thyroid adenoma from a cat with hyperthyroidism. This is a benign but functional tumour (top half); it is well-demarcated from the adjacent thyroid tissue (bottom half) and still forms some follicles containing colloid (pale to bright pink). Tumour cells have minimal atypia and mitotic figures are rare to absent. The production of thyroid hormones is no longer regulated as it should be however, hence the concurrent changes in thyroid stimulating hormone (TSH) and thyrotropin releasing hormone (TRH) as the normal feedback loop is broken.

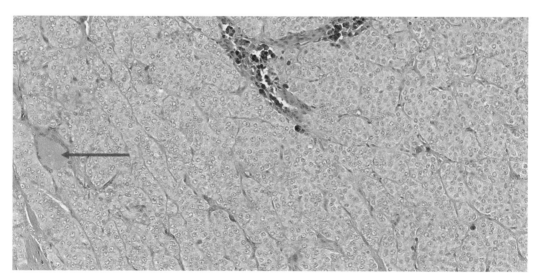

Figure 6.6b Thyroid carcinoma from a dog, and which has a solid growth pattern. There is cellular and nuclear atypia, with some mitotic activity. There is little to no attempt at follicle formation (this photo shows one follicle highlighted by the red arrow, which may even have been pre-existing, but I had to hunt around to find it). These tumours tend to be non-functional, that is, the dogs do not develop hyperthyroidism – I often wonder if they should be hypothyroid, but presumably there is some functional reserve.

Some *changes can be seen at the cellular level*. Neoplastic cells may demonstrate various forms of ana-plasia (cellular atypia), particularly if malignant; they may demonstrate variation in size and shape, and sometimes bizarre giant cells can be seen. Anisocytosis is variation in cellular size. Tumour cells may lose characteristic features such as the cytoplasmic granules seen in mast cells (Figure 6.7). They may have notably basophilic cytoplasm as a result of large numbers of ribosomes – these are needed for rapid cell growth and frequent cell division.

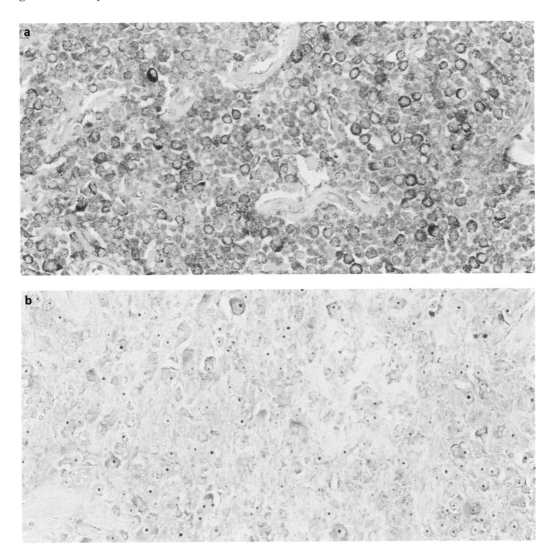

Figure 6.7 Two canine MCTs, stained with Giemsa to demonstrate the cytoplasmic granules characteristic of mast cells. The first (a) is a well-granulated mast cell population while the second (b) is poorly granulated, that is, the tumour cells have lost one of their characteristic features.

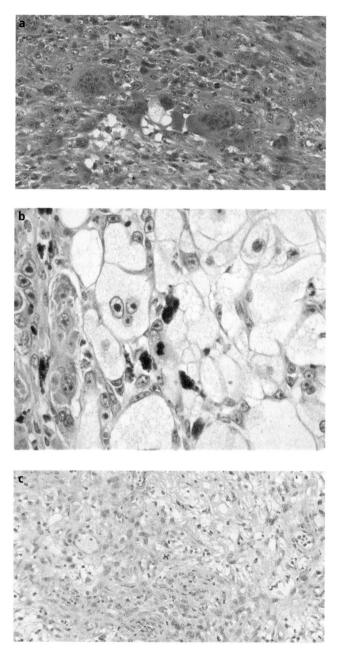

Figure 6.8 Neoplasms demonstrating changes at the nuclear and cellular level. (a) Multi-nucleate cells, with prominent nucleoli (poorly differentiated sarcoma of soft tissues, cat). (b) Bi- and multi-nucleate cells, bizarre nuclei, marginated chromatin, prominent nucleoli, marked anisocytosis and anisokaryosis (poorly melanized melanoma, balloon cell type, haired skin of a dog). (c) 'X marks the spot'. An example of an abnormal mitotic figure, a definite indication of malignancy, poorly differentiated neoplasm in the skin of a dog, confirmed by IHC to be a carcinoma (positive for pancytokeratin), but the primary origin was never determined.

At the nuclear level, there may be variation is size (anisokaryosis), number (bi- and multi-nucleate cells – Figure 6.8a and b), shape, chromatin distribution, nucleolar size and number. Nuclei may be hyperchromatic due to an increased amount of DNA content, or they may be disproportionally large compared to the cell, resulting in an increased nuclear:cytoplasmic ratio. Some nuclei may have clumped and/or marginated chromatin, different to their non-neoplastic counterparts. Increased numbers of mitotic figures, and particularly any abnormal mitotic figures would also be features to look for (Figure 6.8c). Pleomorphism describes variability in size, shape or staining of cells and/or their nuclei.

Other features consistent with or suggestive of malignancy would include evidence of lymphovascular invasion and necrosis within parts of the tumour (Figure 6.9). However, some features such as nuclear pleomorphism should be interpreted in conjunction with knowledge of that particular neoplasm and the prognostic significance or otherwise – again, this is where the experience and knowledge of the pathologist comes into play (Figure 6.10).

Inflammatory and neoplastic pathology

Differentiating between inflammatory and neoplastic pathology is not always as easy as you might think. This is because some of the features discussed above are not specific to neoplasia, but can be seen in other non-neoplastic pathologies, such as with chronic inflammation, irritation or trauma, and reactive or regenerative processes. I have tried to illustrate this with some specific examples below.

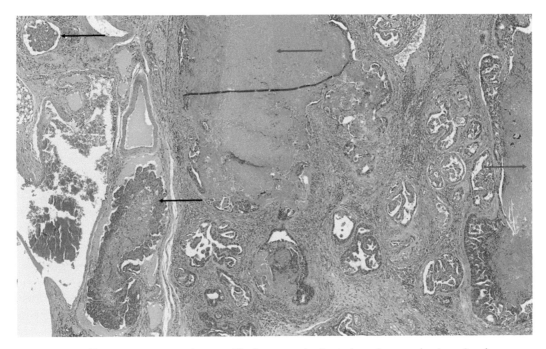

Figure 6.9 Feline mammary carcinoma. Black arrows indicate lymphovascular invasion by the neoplastic cells, red arrows highlight the presence of necrosis. Both are indicators of malignancy in this case.

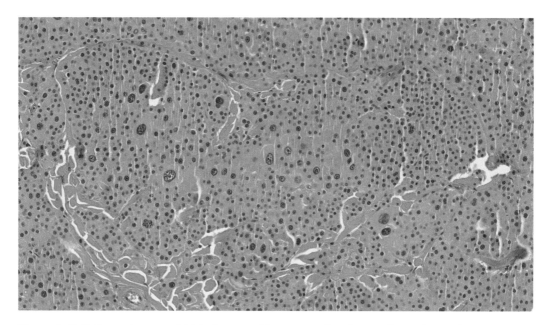

Figure 6.10 Feline cutaneous MCT, pleomorphic mastocytic subtype. Note the nuclear pleomorphism visible even at low power. In these tumours, this has not shown to correlate with prognosis (depending on the precise study you read).

Mast cell tumours

An individual, well-differentiated, well-granulated neoplastic mast cell is indistinguishable from a normal resident mast cell (present in many tissues) or even from a reactive mast cell seen as part of an inflammatory process (Figure 6.11). The key is the growth pattern; normal or reactive mast cells should be present as individual cells, while neoplastic mast cells tend to form aggregates or clusters. We tend to use a cut-off of three or more mast cells in a cluster as a cause for concern, but this is solely based on the criteria in Weishaar et al. (2014), where they propose a classification system for evaluating lymph nodes for evidence of metastatic disease; in this study they looked at the number of, distribution of, and architectural disruption by nodal mast cells and corresponded this to the likelihood of it being metastatic disease.

Obviously when large numbers of mast cells are forming a distinct mass, it is easy to diagnose a neoplastic process – the challenge comes when assessing smaller numbers of mast cells at or close to surgical margins, as you expect to see non-neoplastic mast cells recruited to the site of a MCT. This is because neoplastic mast cells and eosinophils release various cytokines and other bioactive mediators which attract non-neoplastic mast cells towards them, so there is likely to be a rim of non-neoplastic mast cells present at the periphery of a MCT. The other challenge comes when examining revised surgical scar lines, as mast cells are a normal part of the healing process and are involved in remodelling of the wound, so they will certainly be present in those tissues also.

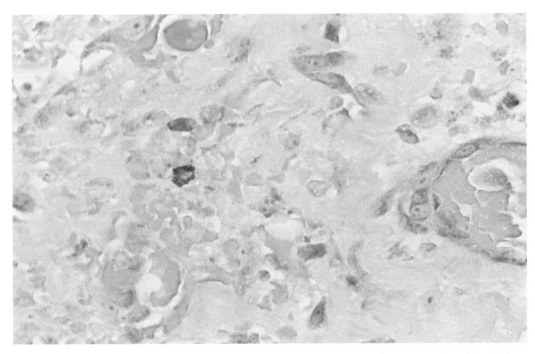

Figure 6.11 Giemsa stain showing a single, well-granulated mast cell. On a single cell basis, it is impossible to determine whether this particular mast cell is reactive or neoplastic and the overall context is vital; in this case, this mast cell was present within an inflammatory lesion.

Rhabdomyosarcoma (sarcoma of skeletal muscle)

Figure 6.12 illustrates a rhabdomyosarcoma from the neck of a dog, which varies in the degree of differentiation in different parts of the tumour. This neoplastic process is compared to an inflammatory one also arising in muscle – a case of masticatory muscle myositis (MMM). These two cases illustrate that some of the changes seen are not necessarily specific to neoplasia and thus they always have to be assessed in context with the other changes present in the section and with the clinical history.

Hepatocellular lesions

We have already looked at benign and malignant hepatocellular tumours. Figure 6.13a shows a higher power view of the benign 'hepatoma', showing the neoplastic cells in more detail. Note there is nuclear pleomorphism, occasional bi-nucleate cells, and often prominent nucleoli. Compare this to the image of a liver biopsy from a dog with a chronic hepatopathy (Figure 6.13b). In the presence of hepatocyte loss, the remaining hepatocytes will attempt to regenerate; the signs of this include variation in nuclear size, bi-nucleate cells and even (if severe enough) mitotic figures. Once again, we see that these changes are not specific to neoplasia and have to be assessed in the wider context – in a case such as this, that would include the clinical presentation, gross appearance (that is, a mass-lesion or diffuse change), and what other histological changes are present in our sections, such as inflammation, fibrosis, biliary proliferation and/or hepatocyte apoptosis/necrosis.

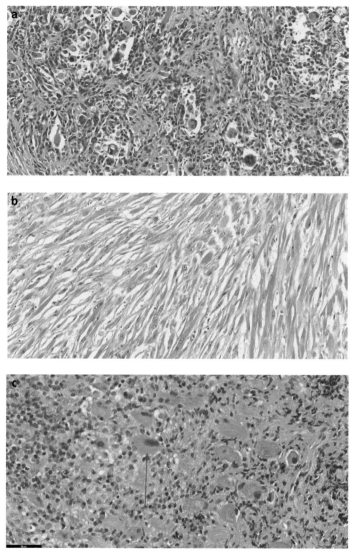

Figure 6.12 A rhabdomyosarcoma arising from the neck musculature of a dog. (a) Note that the tumour cells vary in size and in shape. Some have larger amounts of cytoplasm which is more eosinophilic (pink) like a normal muscle cell, while other cells have smaller amounts of cytoplasm which is more basophilic (blue). Some cells have multiple nuclei, and the nuclei also vary in size and shape. (b) This is a different area of the same tumour. In this field, the neoplastic cells look more like elongated skeletal muscle cells, although they still demonstrate a degree of cellular and nuclear atypia. (c) For comparison, this image is of skeletal muscle from a case of MMM, also from a dog (temporal muscle). These muscle cells are not neoplastic, they are in fact attempting to regenerate – they have smaller amounts of more basophilic cytoplasm and vary in size and shape. They also may have multiple nuclei (red arrow), some with prominent nucleoli. This illustrates that some of these changes are not necessarily specific to neoplasia and thus they always have to be assessed in context with the other changes present in the section and with the clinical history.

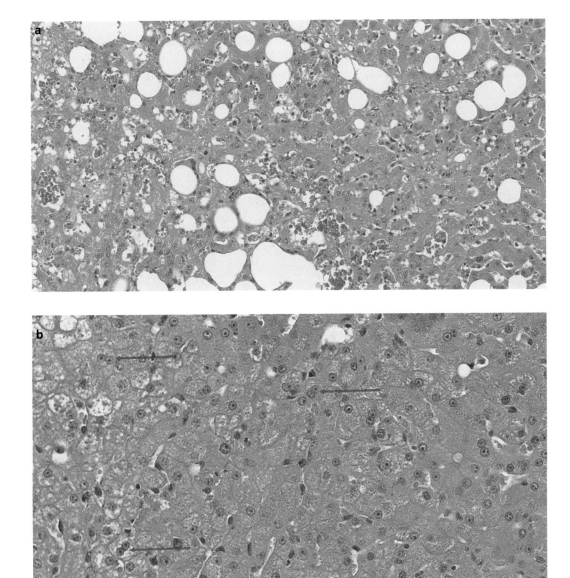

Figure 6.13 Liver biopsies. (a) From a dog with a benign 'hepatoma', demonstrating features such as nuclear pleomorphism, occasional bi-nucleate cells, and often prominent nucleoli, together with an absence of lobular architecture such as cords and sinusoids. (b) From a dog with chronic hepatopathy. In the presence of hepatocyte loss, the remaining hepatocytes will attempt to regenerate and may demonstrate features including variation in nuclear size, bi-nucleate cells (red arrows) and mitotic figures.

Lymph nodes: reactive hyperplasia versus lymphoma

We have already looked at some of the challenges of differentiating some forms of lymphoma from reactive lymphoid hyperplasia, in Chapter 3, when we discussed the pros and cons of different biopsy types. In that chapter, we looked at the importance of the overall architecture of the lymph node in trying to reach a diagnosis. In Chapter 5, in the section on immunohistochemistry, we also looked at the benefits of immunophenotyping – as this helps us to determine whether a lymphoid population is a mixture of B-cells and T-cells, or all of the same immunophenotype; this also helps us to assess the architecture of the lymph node and whether it is consistent with a reactive hyperplasia, or an emerging lymphoma. Sometimes we still need further testing in the form of PARR, to determine whether lymphocytes have arisen from a single clone or multiple.

We sometimes need these adjunctive tests because the cellular and nuclear features of reactive lymphocytes and neoplastic ones often overlap with one another (Figure 6.14). Sometimes even the architectural features of a lymph node are such that we are unable to make a confident diagnosis, such as when we see 'atypical' hyperplasia of lymph nodes – one good example of this is the now well-recognized atypical lymphoid hyperplasia presenting as a generalized lymphadenomegaly, seen as a side effect with methimazole administration for feline hyperthyroidism (Niessen et al., 2007).

Fibroblasts: reactive or neoplastic?

This one is a classic pathologist's conundrum. There is no single feature or stain that will differentiate between a reactive fibroblast and a neoplastic one, and so we are often heavily reliant on other features to

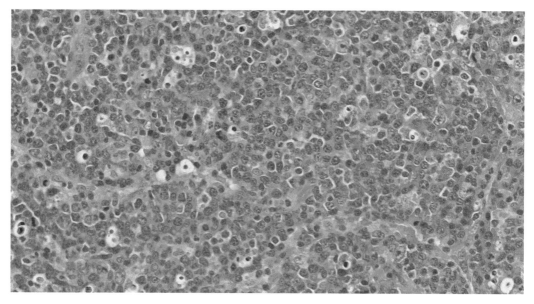

Figure 6.14 Image taken from a submandibular lymph node, from a young dog with localized lymphadenopathy. In this particular region of the lymph node, there was loss of normal architecture and although the lymphocyte population is mixed, there is a predominance of larger lymphoid cells, some demonstrating mitotic activity. We overall favoured a reactive hyperplasia, although this one carried a health warning!

help us decide. These include the cellularity of a lesion, the overall growth pattern (Are there streams and bundles, haphazard arrangement, relationship to other features?) and presentation (Is it a mass? Is there a history of trauma?), whether there is organization or evidence of maturation (granulation tissues), and what other cells and processes are present in the lesion, for example ulceration, necrosis (and where), inflammatory cells, their types and distribution. Even so, sometimes we cannot be 100% confident with certain cases, and distinguishing between a low-grade, inflamed soft tissue sarcoma, and a reactive and inflammatory lesion, such as scar tissue arising in fat or muscle, can be impossible. Similarly, it can be very challenging to confidently differentiate between residual neoplastic tissues and florid scar tissue if revision surgery for a sarcoma is performed. Again, sometimes the clinical history can provide essential information or clues to help us shift in favour of a neoplastic or reactive process, so it is important that it is provided.

Figure 6.15 shows granulation tissue. The blue arrow indicates the ulcerated surface, that is, a reason for why there might be a reactive change in the underlying tissues. The black arrow shows more densely cellular areas (immature) of granulation tissues where fibroblasts are likely to look very 'reactive', because they are immediately underneath the area of ulceration and injury. The green arrow indicates less cellular (more mature) areas further away from the ulcerated surface. This is the expected pattern of maturation seen in granulation tissues and is an appropriate response. The red arrows pick out the regular-spacing of blood vessels often seen in granulation tissues; blood vessels of similar size and in similar orientation within the tissue, perpendicular to the fibroblasts in between. Fibroblasts are also typically neatly arranged in parallel to one another, and there should be some stroma present. Fibroblasts in the more mature areas should also appear less 'reactive'. These are all the types of features a histopathologist might look for when differentiating between reactive fibroplasia and a spindle cell sarcoma, because the nuclear and cellular features alone may not be sufficient.

Figure 6.16 provides some examples to help illustrate some of the challenges we can face with fibroblasts. One should bear in mind that cytologists typically only have cellular and nuclear features to go by,

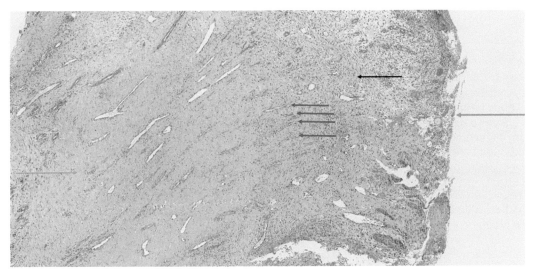

Figure 6.15 Area of granulation tissue proliferation and some of the features a pathologist might look for to differentiate between granulation tissue and a low-grade sarcoma.

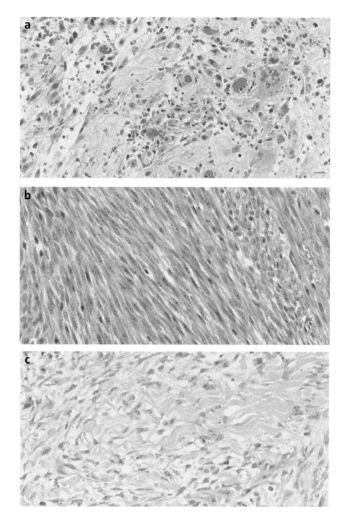

Figure 6.16 (a) Reactive fibroblasts at high-power magnification; note the variation in nuclear size, often large nuclei and prominent nucleoli, the increased nuclear:cytoplasmic ratio, slightly basophilic cytoplasm and variation in cell shape. Low numbers of mitotic figures might also be seen. The fibroblasts are very haphazardly arranged within the tissues. These are all features which might otherwise suggest malignancy, but in this case, they are part of the normal fibroblast response to inflammation or other form of injury. (b) Fibroblasts from a low-grade fibrosarcoma, from the tail of a cat. On an individual cell basis, they are fairly bland, particularly when compared to the reactive fibroblasts in the image above. They have large nuclei but there is little variation in nuclear size or shape, with sometimes prominent nucleoli and occasional mitotic figures. But the lesion presented as a mass, was moderately cellular throughout, with no maturation and little associated inflammation, and fibroblasts were arranged in interlacing bundles and streams (ironically more 'organized' than the fibroblasts in the reactive lesion above), with little to no stroma. (c) What about these cells? Fibroblasts taken from the edge of a sarcoma, but also associated with reactive fibroplasia, ulceration and inflammation elsewhere. Mitotic figures are noted, together with anisokaryosis and prominent nucleoli.

without any of the architectural features to help guide the decision-making process – which is often why cases like this yield the result of 'mesenchymal cell proliferation', which is completely understandable, if sometimes frustrating for the clinician.

Self-assessment: quick fire quiz

1. Which of the following neoplasms is considered benign?
   a Hepatocellular carcinoma
   b Liposarcoma
   c Haemangioma
   d Rhabdomyosarcoma
2. Which of the following characteristics is considered the definitive criterion for malignancy?
   a Frequent metastasis
   b Capsule often present
   c Normal appearing mitotic figures
   d Well-differentiated appearance
3. Which of the following is INCORRECT?
   a Neoplasm means 'new growth'
   b Cancer means 'crab'
   c Metastasis means 'change of place'
   d Tumour means 'neoplastic'
4. Which of the following can be considered a hallmark of differentiation?
   a Loss of normal tissue architecture
   b Hypertrophy
   c Inflammation
   d Presence of portal tracts
5. Which of the following is a cellular feature?
   a Anisokaryosis
   b Multinucleation
   c Abnormal mitotic figures
   d Anisocytosis

The answers are available on page 184.

Oncology: histological descriptions, grading of neoplasms and additional prognostication

7

Introduction

In this chapter, we will take a look at histological descriptions of neoplasms to better understand what the pathologist is seeing on the slide. We will also look at some of the histological grading systems currently available for some tumours, with their various pros and cons and what they can tell us in terms of prognosis. Finally, we will look at some of the additional prognostic tests which are available, in particular for MCTs and melanocytic neoplasms.

Histological descriptions of neoplasms

There is no one way of describing lesions in pathology, and pathologists each have their own individual styles to some extent. However, there are features which are often incorporated into the description of a neoplastic process, typically the features we have already discussed in Chapter 6. One way to describe a tumour is to use the 'seven sentence approach'.

Sentence 1 Low power – location/tissue affected, description of mass and growth pattern

These **tissues** are occupied and expanded by a **size** (small, medium, large), **cellularity** (densely, moderately cellular), **infiltration** (infiltrative, expansile, encapsulated, unencapsulated, pseudo-encapsulated), **other** (well-demarcated, poorly demarcated, wedge-shaped, multi-lobular) neoplastic mass.

Some examples:

- The dermis has been focally expanded by a densely cellular, multi-lobular, well-demarcated but unencapsulated neoplastic mass.
- The dermis and subcutis are occupied and expanded by a large, roughly spherical, unencapsulated, well-demarcated but infiltrative and densely cellular neoplastic mass, which extends up to the dermal-epidermal junction and is associated with focal areas of epidermal ulceration.
- The liver parenchyma is occupied, expanded and somewhat effaced by a poorly demarcated, infiltrative, unencapsulated, moderately cellular, oedematous and multilobulated neoplastic mass.

Sentence 2 Tumour cell arrangement – growth pattern of the tumour cells, stroma

Tumour cells are **arranged in** (sheets, cords, streams, bundles, nests, islands, tubules, acini, packets, whorls) and are **supported by (describe stroma)**, extending from the surface deep into the underlying submucosa.

Some examples:

- The tumour cells are arranged in clusters, aggregates, or variably sized and shaped tubules and nests, supported by a moderate amount of fibrous to slightly myxoid stroma.
- Tumour cells are arranged in packets or lobules, sometimes surrounding variably sized spaces filled with pale, eosinophilic fluid, or with central areas of cells with pyknotic or karyolytic nuclei and brightly eosinophilic cytoplasm (necrosis); tumour cells are supported by a fine, fibrovascular network.
- The tumour cells are arranged in sheets and in places are forming cords; they are supported by a fine fibrovascular stroma and in most fields are infiltrating between and separating pre-existing dermal collagen fibre bundles, adipocytes, glands and blood vessels.

Sentence 3 The tumour cells, their cytoplasm and their cell borders

Cell size/shape, amount of cytoplasm and features such as colour, vacuoles or granularity, pigment, and the cell margins.

The tumour cells are **shape** (round, ovoid, polypoid, cuboidal, angular, columnar, polygonal, elongated, spindle-shaped), with a (small, moderate, large) **amount** of (eosinophilic, basophilic, homogenous, granular, fibrillary, pale staining, floccular, vacuolated) **cytoplasm** that has (well-defined, poorly defined, indistinct) **margins** and **contains** (numerous Giemsa-positive granules – for example, MCT, finely granular brown pigment – for example, melanoma)

Some examples:

- The tumour cells are medium to large and polygonal, cuboidal to columnar in shape, with moderate amounts of sometimes granular or vacuolated, brightly eosinophilic cytoplasm and distinct cell borders; occasional tumour cells contain moderate amounts of brown pigment granules within their cytoplasm.
- The tumour cells are polygonal or elongated, and medium-sized, with small to moderate amounts of finely granular, eosinophilic and occasionally vacuolated cytoplasm with sometimes indistinct margins.
- The tumour cells are round, ovoid or polygonal, with a moderate amount of vacuolated eosinophilic cytoplasm that has well-defined margins and sometimes contains numerous small granules (Giemsa positive).

Sentence 4 Nucleus

Nuclei are **size** (large, small), **location** (central, paracentral, eccentric) and **shape** (ovoid, round, C-shaped, bean-shaped, elongated, indented), with (densely packed, finely granular, reticulated, sparse, largely marginated, partially marginated) **chromatin** and **number** of (small, prominent, central, eccentric, barely detectable, inobtrusive, not visible?) deeply eosinophilic **nucleoli**.

Some examples:

- The nuclei are large, ovoid or elongated, variably located within the cells, and have moderately dense, granular chromatin and single, inconspicuous, deeply eosinophilic, mostly paracentral nucleoli.
- The nuclei are moderately sized to large, round, ovoid or very occasionally indented and are eccentric or paracentral; they contain finely stippled, partially marginated chromatin and 1, 2 or occasionally 3, deeply eosinophilic and occasionally large nucleoli which can be located central, paracentral or eccentric within the nucleus.
- Tumour nuclei are medium to large, paracentral or eccentric and round to ovoid, with small amounts of finely stippled, partially marginated chromatin and 1–2, often large, prominent nucleoli.

Sentence 5 Cellular and nuclear size, variation and mitotic figures

There is (mild, moderate, marked) **anisokaryosis** (with occasional large, giant cells, multi-nucleated) and **mitotic figures** (are not noted, average per high-power field (400×) or give range, with some bizarre appearances).

An example:

- There is moderate to marked anisokaryosis and moderate anisocytosis, with occasional bi- and multi-nucleate cells and 23 mitotic figures seen in 10 HPFs (400×; 2.37 mm^2), some of which have a bizarre appearance.

Sentence 6 Extras

Note, for example, presence of inflammation, epidermal ulceration, necrosis, oedema, congestion, lymphoid invasion and other cells evident.

Some examples:

- There is extensive, central epidermal ulceration and erosion overlying the mass, with clear spaces superficially (oedema).
- The mass is associated with aggregates of lymphoid cells scattered throughout, as well as multifocal, sometimes locally extensive areas of necrosis.
- There are occasional clusters of neoplastic cells present within vessels at the periphery.
- Associated apocrine glands are markedly dilated.

Sentence 7 Margins

- The tumour appears separated from the lateral and deep margins in the sections examined; measurements.

Although the precise format used will vary between laboratories, the report should also contain a diagnosis and a comment, as a minimum. The diagnosis should clearly specify the tumour type (as far as possible), the histological grade if applicable and the location. The comment will typically include the diagnosis, and details regarding margins if appropriate (that is, if an excisional rather than incisional sample was submitted), the grade (where applicable), and the expected clinical behaviour for a neoplasm of that type. It may include advice regarding staging and/or monitoring for local recurrence. If there are additional tests which may either aid further diagnosis (for example, IHC for a poorly differentiated neoplasm) or prognosis (Ki67 scoring, immunophenotyping) then these will also be discussed in the comments. Some pathologists have moved away from giving a prognosis in recent years, as after consultation with oncologists it was felt this was not always helpful – the opinion being that a true and accurate prognosis is highly individual and depends not only on histological findings but also on many other factors which the pathologist is often not privy too – such as clinical features, the client, the animal and concurrent conditions, financial situations, and availability of therapeutic options.

Different tumour types were covered in Chapter 5, in the section on immunohistochemistry, with regard to classifying sarcomas, carcinomas and round cell tumours. That section also covers some of the uses of immunohistochemistry in diagnosis and also prognostication, including immunophenotyping of lymphomas, Ki67 and MCM7 scoring of MCTs, and KIT pattern assessment.

Histological grading systems

Avallone et al.'s (2021) excellent review on this topic, 'Review of histological grading systems in veterinary medicine', is well worth a read.

This chapter will now cover some of the more commonly used grading systems. There are new ones being published all the time – bear in mind, however, that not all are equally validated or useful. Some have a very poor evidence base or have a lack of detailed instructions in the materials and methods section meaning that pathologists struggle to apply them to their own cases. It is important for pathologists and oncologists to be aware of the limitations of grading, including sometimes a lack of validation studies or clear prognostic relevance. We have already touched on the challenges of grading tumours based on only incisional biopsies, in Chapter 3 under 'Different types of biopsies, their pros and cons'. Other problems we may encounter with published grading systems is a lack of clarity over the field size used to calculate mitotic count and poor consistency between studies, meaning results cannot be compared. This is something that has recently been recognized and as such there are movements to try and improve on the situation. It is suggested you refer to the Veterinary Canine Guidelines and Protocols website for more detail (www.vcgp.org/).

Remember also that studies look at a population of animals with a given neoplasm, and that our patients are individuals. Not every patient can be the median, some will inevitably survive for shorter or longer than the median survival time quoted in any particular study and there will always be outliers.

Canine cutaneous mast cell tumours

The combination of the high incidence of mast cell tumours (MCTs), their highly variable and potentially fatal biological behaviour and their potential for paraneoplastic effects all mean that the accurate prognostication of MCTs is vital. The single most valuable prognostic factor is still the histological grade. There are several grading systems, which are discussed further below, but note that these are only validated for cutaneous MCTs and should not be applied in primarily subcutaneous, mucosal or visceral MCTs. The grading systems are validated for primary tumours only, and the prognostic significance of grading a recurrent MCT is currently also unknown. Grading of small pre-treatment incisional biopsies is becoming more widely performed, but please note that this does result in underestimation of the histological grade in a minority of cases.

There are actually two different three-tier systems for histological grading of canine cutaneous MCTs, Bostock in 1973 and Patnaik in 1984, but unfortunately, they grade MCTs in the opposite order to one another. Hence a well-differentiated MCT would be a grade I Patnaik but a grade III Bostock, and a poorly differentiated MCT would be a grade III Patnaik but a grade I Bostock. Also, both systems use slightly differing grading criteria; Bostock uses nuclear:cytoplasmic ratio (N:C), mitotic rate, tumour cellularity and the presence of granules, while Patnaik uses cell morphology, mitotic rate, tumour cellularity, tumour extent and stromal reaction (see Table 7.1). Fortunately, most pathologists use the Patnaik grading system and also state whether the tumour is well-differentiated, of intermediate differentiation or poorly differentiated, in addition to assigning a numerical grade, thus hopefully avoiding confusion!

However, there are problems with the Patnaik system, one of which being a predominance of grade II (intermediate-grade) tumours. Some of these grade II tumours are biologically aggressive but are not distinguished as such, because the Patnaik system unfortunately has some grade III criteria that exclude these aggressive MCTs from the higher category. Another problem is the criteria using any extension of neoplastic mast cells below the dermis and adnexa and into the subcutis; often this is the criterion which pushes an otherwise low-grade MCT towards being classified as a grade II rather than a grade I.

With both of these factors at play, it is little wonder that grade II encompasses up to 59% of all MCTs, and that this is a biologically diverse group of tumours. This consequently means that all grade II tumours have historically had to be regarded as potentially malignant and this makes it difficult to predict what additional therapy, if any, should be given to these dogs. Metastatic spread is reported to occur in 5–22% of grade II MCTs, with local recurrence occurring in 5–11%. In the original study by Patnaik, 43%

of MCT tumours were given a grade II, and of those 56% of the patients were dead due to the MCT at 1500 days (5 years). Therefore, grading a MCT as a grade II really is of little prognostic value, since these dogs have almost a 50 : 50 chance of dying due to their tumour within 5 years.

A two-tier grading system was subsequently suggested (Kiupel et al., 2011), which avoided the use of tumour depth altogether and aimed to divide the intermediate-grade II tumours into two groups, low grade or high grade (grade I Patnaik tumours are always low grade with Kiupel, and grade III Patnaik tumours are always high grade). Having two tiers rather than three also avoids the tendency of pathologists (who are only human after all!) to 'sit on the fence' and call tumours intermediate grade. The criteria are also, for the main part, objective rather than subjective, which helps to mitigate inter-pathologist variation. The two-tier system uses a mitotic count greater than 7 per 10 HPFs (400×), together with karyomegaly (large nuclear size) and the presence of multi-nucleate cells (three or more nuclei per cell) and/or bizarre nuclei. Tumours are categorized as either low grade or high grade (see Table 7.1). According to this system, the majority of canine cutaneous MCTs are low grade. Low-grade MCTs have a lower rate of recurrence, metastasis and tumour-related death than high-grade MCTs using this system.

Some studies have suggested that within the Kiupel high-grade group of MCTs, there is still a difference between Patnaik grade II and grade III tumours. Because of this, and the fact that oncologists and clinicians are still most familiar with the Patnaik system, both grading systems are frequently used when reporting routine diagnostic cases.

Some groups have attempted to use mitotic count alone as a prognostic indicator, but unfortunately this method still misses some of the biologically aggressive tumours. Cut-off values for distinguishing high-grade MCTs vary between studies from 5 to 10 mitotic figures per 10 HPFs, which in a way illustrates how unreliable mitotic index is as a sole prognostic indicator.

The majority of MCTs originate in the dermis and extend into the subcutis, but there is a subset that is restricted to the subcutaneous fat and are classified as a subtype in their own right – subcutaneous MCTs. This is determined on the basis of location within the subcutaneous tissue and no invasion of the dermis, although multifocal extension of low numbers of mast cells around the base of hair follicles or mast cells infiltrating the underlying panniculus musculature is allowed, as long as the bulk of the tumour is within the subcutaneous tissue. There is no supporting evidence for the usefulness of grading these tumours with any of the cutaneous grading systems, but a few studies have looked at the prognostication of subcutaneous MCTs as a separate entity. Tumours should be assessed based on the growth pattern, presence of multinucleation (defined as more than 1 nuclei per cell, present if there was at least 1 multinucleated cell in 10 HPFs [400×]), and the mitotic count. The strongest effect on clinical outcome appears to be mitotic activity. Subcutaneous tumours are more effectively controlled by surgery alone than their cutaneous counterparts. Surgery is curative for the majority of these tumours.

Feline cutaneous mast cell tumours

A two-tier histological grading system has been proposed for feline cutaneous MCTs also (Sabattini and Bettini, 2019), although further validation is still needed. In our own studies (Melville et al., 2015), we also found that the feature with the best prognostic value was still the mitotic count, and we found the same cut-off value of 5 per 10 HPFs (400×). However, we also found there was a huge range of mitotic activity in both clinically benign MCTs and those which ultimately resulted in the death of the cat.

Table 7.1 Comparison of grading systems

MCT type	Patnaik grade and criteria		Bostock grade and criteria		Two-tier (Kiupel) and criteria	
Well-differentiated	I	Located in dermis Low cellularity Round, monomorphic cells Distinct cell boundaries Medium-sized granules Round nucleus No mitoses	III	Well-defined cell boundaries Regular, spherical nucleus N : C ratio <0.55 MFs extremely rare	Low	Absence of any of the criteria below
Intermediate	II	Located in dermis and subcutis Moderate to high cellularity Round to ovoid, some pleomorphism Scattered spindle and giant cells Distinct cell boundaries Fine granules Round to indented nuclei Occasionally binucleated Mitoses rare (0–2/HPF)	II	Indistinct cell boundaries N : C ratio 0.55–0.7 Cells more pleomorphic Nuclei more often indented MFs infrequent Cells closely packed	High	Any one of the following: a. at least 7 MFs in 10 HPFs b. at least 3 multinucleate cells (3+ nuclei) in 10 HPFs c. at least 3 bizarre nuclei in 10 HPFs d. karyomegaly
Poorly differentiated	III	Infiltrates subcutis and deeper High cellularity Round, ovoid, spindloid Pleomorphic cells Indistinct cell boundaries Fine granules or none Indented or vesiculated nuclei with 1+ nucleoli Multinucleated cells Mitoses common (3–6/HPF)	I	Highly cellular, more densely packed Indistinct cell boundaries Irregular shaped nuclei N : C ratio >0.7 MFs can be very frequent High degree cellular pleomorphism Bizarre multinucleated giant cells		

The histological subtype (Figure 7.1) and the presence of multiple tumours in the same individual have not been shown to be of prognostic significance. However, we do always warn that cutaneous lesions may represent metastatic spread of a primary visceral MCT, particularly if multiple such skin masses are present.

High-grade tumours have a mitotic count of more than 5 per 10 HPFs, plus at least two of the following features: tumour diameter of greater than 1.5 cm, nuclear pleomorphism and nucleolar prominence / chromatin clusters. One issue with this system is that we do not always know the diameter of the tumour, since we receive it fixed and sometimes only parts. Irregular nuclear shape and nucleolar prominence are also both subjective features.

Canine soft tissue sarcoma (STS, tumours of soft tissues, soft tissue tumours)

This histological grading system is actually based on the human system (Trojani et al., 1984), however, the two groups of tumours in these two species are not entirely the same, with some entities excluded or included from one set or the other (Box 7.1). Studies into these tumours sometimes lack specific diagnoses – in the absence of extensive IHC characterization it can be difficult to differentiate between the different types of STS, and given that the biological behaviour is the same regardless of the specific diagnosis, the cost of such IHC is often difficult to justify. Sometimes studies include benign tumours. Overall, this means that the application of the canine grading system is fairly different to the approach in humans, even though we have 'borrowed' their system.

In dogs, the grading system is typically applied to fibrosarcoma, nerve sheath tumours, perivascular wall tumours and undifferentiated pleomorphic sarcoma, but generally not to rhabdomyosacoma or leiomyosarcoma (although this varies), and definitely not for histiocytic sarcoma. It is also not validated for canine haemangiosarcoma or for use in other species.

Box 7.1 Entities included in the category 'soft tissue sarcoma' – human and canine.

HUMAN (Trojani et al., 1985)
- Liposarcoma
- Tendosynovial sarcoma
- Malignant fibrous histocytosis
- Neurosarcoma
- Rhabdomyosarcoma
- Fibrosarcoma
- Haemangiopericytoma
- Leiomyosarcoma
- Clear-cell sarcoma
- Haemangiosarcoma
- Epithelioid sarcoma
- Alveolar soft-part sarcoma
- Extraosseous osteogenic sarcoma
- Undifferentiated sarcoma

CANINE (Dennis et al., 2011)
- Fibrosarcoma, including keloidal
- Myxosarcoma
- Liposarcoma
- Perivascular wall tumours
- (peripheral) nerve sheath tumour
- Pleomorphic sarcoma
- Mesenchymoma
- ? Leiomyosarcoma
- ? Rhabdomyosarcoma

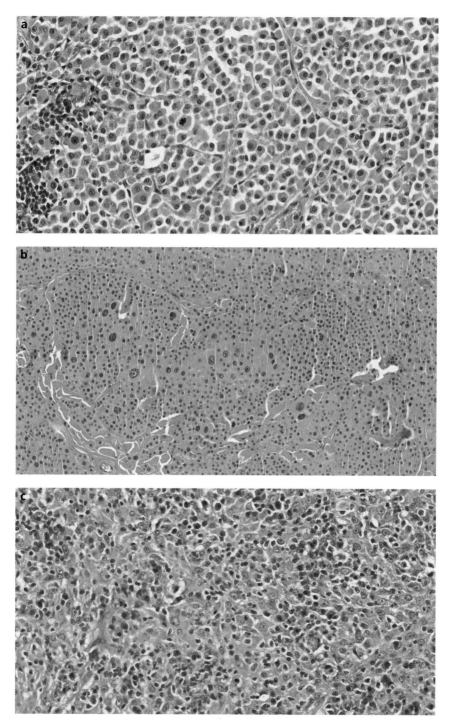

Figure 7.1 Different histological subtypes of feline cutaneous MCTs: (a) well-differentiated mastocytic; (b) pleomorphic mastocytic; (c) atypical (formerly known as histiocytic).

Table 7.2 Criteria used when grading a canine soft tissue sarcoma. Note that 'differentiation score' is entirely subjective and poorly defined for canine tumours

Mitotic score	Number of mitoses per 10 HPFs (400×)
1	0–9
2	10–19
3	More than 19
Tumour necrosis score	Necrosis as % of tumour area
0	No necrosis
1	Less than or equal to 50% necrosis
2	More than 50% necrosis
Differentiation score	
1	
2	
3	
HISTOLOGICAL GRADE	TOTAL SCORE
I (low)	Equal to or less than 3
II (intermediate)	4–5
III (high)	6 or more

The differentiation score is a subjective criterion; when looking at the Trojani paper for humans, they state the following:

- Score 1: sarcomas closely resembling normal adult mesenchymal tissue (well-differentiated liposarcoma, leiomyosarcoma). These tumours are typically not included in the canine STS group.
- Score 2: sarcomas for which the histological typing is certain.
- Score 3: embryonal sarcomas, undifferentiated sarcomas and sarcomas of doubtful tumour type.

Looking at studies on canine STS, the grade of tumour is associated with overall survival in some studies, and with local recurrence, but consistent studies on the impact of grade on the risk of metastatic spread are somewhat lacking. In McSporran (2009) for example, clean margins were predictive for tumour free survival times. But note that the grade was predictive of local recurrence, not for overall patient survival. This study found that clean histological margins were the most important prognostic factor for local recurrence – none of the completely excised tumours in their study with follow-up data available had any evidence of local recurrence. The grade was predictive of recurrence but only for those marginally excised tumours and for those tumours, the time to recurrence significantly varied between grades, and time to local recurrence was inversely related to the tumour grade overall.

Dennis et al. (2011) is an excellent review of canine STS and grading – overall, metastatic disease is rare to infrequent in these tumours, although the likelihood of metastatic disease appears to increase with grade. Local recurrence is dependent on margins, and again, increases in frequency with the grade of the tumour.

The same grading system has also been applied to visceral, non-angiomatous sarcomas in dogs (Linden et al., 2019), that is, sarcomas which are not haemangiosarcoma, arising from sites such as the spleen and intestines. In this study, the most common tumour locations were the spleen (47.6%) and small intestine (23.8%). The local recurrence rate was low (4.7%). Metastasis was present at the time of surgery in 23.8%, and the overall metastatic rate was 40.4%. A mitotic count of more than or equal to 9 was associated with significantly shorter median survival time (MST 269 days) compared with a mitotic count of less than 9 (MST not reached). The MST for grade I tumours was not reached, was 589 days for grade II and 158 days for grade III. Dogs with grade III tumours were more likely to develop metastatic disease. Neither location of the primary tumour nor the histologic subtype was associated with survival time. This study was based retrospectively on a relatively small group of tumours and further work is needed to validate this grading of visceral sarcomas.

Feline STS (including feline injection site sarcoma)

The canine (and human) grading system has also been applied to feline injection site sarcomas (FISS) specifically, in several studies. One study did not have outcome data (Couto et al., 2002) but another did have outcome, in terms of recurrence and mortality (Porcellato et al., 2017). Porcellato found two factors were prognostic in terms of local recurrence – the size of tumour and the mitotic count, which was also prognostic in relation to mortality – but not the grade. They also found mitotic count was a good predictor of mortality, reporting median disease-free interval and medial survival times – for the no local recurrence group, note that there were no deaths due to tumour-related disease, with a good follow-up period. They also found no association between the completeness of surgical margins and recurrence risk.

Our own study (Dobromylskyj et al., 2021) proposed a modified grading system for feline cutaneous and STSs, which included FISS (since it is often difficult to prove whether a particular tumour is a FISS or not). We changed the subjective criterion of differentiation for a factor which we found to be significant when analysed individually, namely the degree of inflammation (Table 7.3). Unfortunately, this is also a somewhat subjective score, but we do at least have evidence to suggest it is significant in these tumours in this species. Drawbacks of the study include the inflammation score being subjective and the relatively small scale. We clearly need a larger scale, preferably prospective study to validate this system, as in this initial study we found a significant association between the histological grade and the survival time. We also hope to use this same cohort in the future to look for other prognostic features.

Lymphoma

Once you start looking in detail at published studies, 'grading' of lymphoma is actually a bit of a nightmare. This is because of the variety of different types (classifications) of lymphoma and the different anatomical sites at which they can arise. It is simply not a homogenous disease. Except for follicular lymphomas, mitotic activity is the key feature we rely on and for which we have an evidence base of sorts. However, even this is complicated by the fact that mitotic count has been calculated in different ways in different studies, at different magnifications, with unspecified field sizes, and number of fields

Table 7.3 **Proposed grading system for feline STSs**

Mitotic score	Number of mitoses per 10 HPFs (400×)
1	0–9
2	10–19
3	More than 19
Tumour necrosis score	**Necrosis as % of tumour area**
0	No necrosis
1	Less than or equal to 50% necrosis
2	More than 50% necrosis
Inflammation score	
1	None, minimal or very mild
2	Mild to moderate
3	Severe
HISTOLOGICAL GRADE	**TOTAL SCORE**
I (low)	Equal to or less than 3
II (intermediate)	4–5
III (high)	6 or more

and in different parts of the mass. This lack of standardization and consistency means findings between different studies often cannot be directly compared. Any association between mitotic count and tumour behaviour/outcome is also often evaluated by 'lumping together' lymphomas of different types within the same study (inconsistently), again leading to inconsistent and somewhat unreliable results – this impacts the apparent prognostic significance of mitotic count and grading of lymphomas, with variable results depending on the study.

There is also a lot of confusion with regards to terminology, and there is a need to separate out clinical behaviour, classification of lymphoma and the histological grade, among oncologists, clinical and anatomical pathologists.

Classification of a lymphoma is the process of giving a name to the specific lymphoma type and will involve multiple features including IHC to determine the immunophenotype(s), for example, diffuse large B-cell lymphoma. It is not the same as grading.

Clinical grading is applied to indicate the likely biological behaviour in an untreated neoplasm, for example, a high-grade lymphoma – but this is not the same as the histological grade. The recommendation has been made that we should use the terms indolent, intermediate and aggressive behaviour to stratify lymphomas by their predicted clinical course, and not to describe the histological grade.

Histological grade is the bit pathologists do (as well as the classification). It has been suggested pathologists use the terms low, intermediate and high grade when talking about the histological grade only.

So, what about histological grading then?

Nearly all of the studies have been performed on lymphomas in dogs and for disease arising in lymph nodes. 'Specific guidelines for histological grading of animal lymphomas that are located in anatomical sites other than lymph nodes have not been established yet and there is no current evidence that grading lymphomas at these sites for example, (alimentary, respiratory, skin) has prognostic relevance' (Avallone et al., 2021: 817). The one exception to this rule might be the canine and feline small cell lymphomas with a low mitotic count arising within the GI tract, which appear to have a better prognosis than large cell lymphomas with a high mitotic count at this site.

The most commonly used grading scheme for lymphoma is the WHO grading scheme (Valli et al., 2002), which has been applied to two large cohorts of dogs with nodal lymphoma (Valli et al., 2011, 2013). It only uses the mitotic count, based on the number of mitoses in one 400× HPF, although the exact method of calculating this number is unclear and there seems to be some disagreement about whether you should count 10 HPFs and use the average, or use the highest number you see in a single HPF.

Box 7.2 Grading system for canine lymphoma

Histological Grade	Mitotic count
Grade I (low)	0–5 / HPF
Grade II (medium)	6–10 / HPF
Grade III (high)	more than 10 / HPF

The same two studies did classify using other features including immunophenotype, maturity of cells, growth pattern (nodular verses diffuse) and nuclear size, but these were not used to determine the grade.

Box 7.3 Nuclear size

Small	less than 1.5 the size of a RBC
Intermediate	1.5–2 times the size of a RBC
Large	more than 2 times the size of a RBC

One of those two studies (Valli et al., 2013, as discussed in Avallone et al., 2021) looked at mitotic count and clinical behaviour: when they divided the cases into the three groups using the cut-off values for grading, it did not correlate with overall survival. But when they divided into two groups instead (using the cut-off of 20 mitotic figures per 400× field) there was good agreement with overall survival. However, this was performed on groups of heterogeneous lymphoma types and some types were only present in low numbers, which may have impacted the survival curves.

Nodular lymphomas (marginal zone, mantle zone, follicular, T-zone)
Note that IHC will be needed to definitively classify some of these, but cell size and growth pattern can be used – these have been found to be associated with a low grade (due to low mitotic count), an indolent clinical course and prolonged survival. In some studies, further grading these types of tumours based on mitotic count did not impact on survival times (that is, grading them is not useful for prognosis), however, there may have been bias in the analysis as marginal and TZLs were grouped together in some studies.

Follicular lymphomas (rare in cats and dogs)

This is a separate grading system based on counting the number of centroblasts in 10 neoplastic follicles and stating the average per one 400× field. Information on the utility of this system is lacking.

Box 7.4 Grading system for canine follicular lymphoma

Histological Grade	Number of centroblasts*
Grade I (low)	0–5 / HPF
Grade II (medium)	6–15 / HPF
Grade III (high)	more than 15 / HPF

*defined as large lymphocytes with moderate amount of cytoplasm, round to oval vesicular nucleus and 2–3 nucleoli often located adjacent to the nuclear membrane, assessed in 10 neoplastic follicles and expressed as number per HPF (area of view not specified).

Canine mammary carcinoma

Based on a human system, this is designed only for epithelial tumours, and so cannot be applied to mammary sarcomas (which are relatively rare). It is a widely used system and there is evidence of prognostic usefulness (Table 7.4).

Table 7.4 Grading system for canine mammary carcinoma

Tubule formation	Score
Formation of tubules in more than 75%	1
10–75%, admixed with areas of solid growth	2
Less than 10%, minimal or no tubule formation	3
Nuclear pleomorphism	**Score**
Uniform or regular small nucleus and occasional nucleoli	1
Moderate degree of variation in nuclear size and shape, hyperchromatic nucleus, presence of nucleoli (can be prominent)	2
Marked variation in nuclear size, hyperchromatic nucleus, often with one or more prominent nucleoli	3
Mitotic count (in 10 HPFs, 400×, 2.37 mm²)	**Score**
0–9	1
10–19	2
20 or more	3
HISTOLOGICAL GRADE	**TOTAL SCORE**
I (low)	3–5
II (medium)	6–7
III (high)	8–9

Grade I tumours (low grade) have the longest survival times compared to grade III, with a lower tendency to metastasize to distant organs and for local recurrence. On the other hand, grade III (high-grade) tumours have the shortest survival times, and a greater metastatic risk. For grade II tumours there is no consistent statistically significant difference in survival times compared to grade I tumours, but grade II tumours do have the ability to spread to regional lymph nodes (but more studies are needed).

Other important prognostic factors include the tumour size, clinical stage, histological subtype, histological evidence of infiltrative tumour growth and lymphovascular invasion, independent of the histological grade.

Feline mammary carcinoma

There are several grading systems advised for use in invasive feline mammary carcinomas, with no strong consensus as to which is preferred. The mitotic-modified Elston–Ellis (MMEE) as per Dagher et al. (2019) is one grading system, which is based on the Elston–Ellis system but with mitotic count cut-offs adjusted for feline tumours (Table 7.5). The Mills system is also available (Mills et al., 2015) and shown in Table 7.6.

Table 7.5 **MMEE system**

TUBULE FORMATION	(% of tumour area)	SCORE
	Majority (>75%)	1
	Moderate (10–75%)	2
	Little or none (<10%)	3
NUCLEAR PLEOMORPHISM		**SCORE**
	Small, regular, uniform	1
	Moderate increase in size, vesiculation, and variability	2
	Vesicular chromatin, marked variation in size and shape	3
MITOTIC COUNT	**per 10 HPFs (40x; 0.625 mm)****	**SCORE**
	0–33	1
	34–66	2
	67 or more	3
TOTAL SCORE	**GRADE**	
3–5	I	Well-differentiated
6–7	II	Moderately differentiated
8–9	III	Poorly differentiated

Notes: ** Note the difference in field size.

Table 7.6 Mills-2015 system

Lymphovascular invasion	absent/present	0/1
Nuclear form*	equal to or less than 5% abnormal	0
	more than 5% abnormal	1
Mitotic count	equal to or less than 33	0
	more than 33	1
Score 0	= low grade	
Score 1–3	= high grade	

Some authors suggest using the two in parallel, and some suggest that the Mills system needs further validation. The MMEE grading system has been significantly associated with overall survival, independent of tumour size and positive nodal stage.

There are other grading systems published, too many to cover all of them here. Some of these types of tumours are less commonly seen in our diagnostic pathology service (canine pulmonary carcinoma, canine gliomas, feline non-ocular melanoma, canine and feline meningioma – based on the histological subtype, canine multi-lobular sarcoma of bone, canine urothelial carcinoma), some have a poor evidence base for their usefulness or simply insufficient detail in publications to allow us to apply the system to our own cases. Remember also that sometimes a sample is not suitable for grading to be applied (too small, too crushed, too much artefact).

Additional prognostication

Canine MCTs

AgNOR

AgNOR (argyrophilic nucleolar organizer regions) are areas within the nucleus associated with proteins involved in ribosomal RNA transcription. The number of AgNORs present within each nucleus is proportional to the rate of cell proliferation or the cell doubling time *in vivo*. AgNORs are detected by a histochemical (silver) stain (Figure 7.2), and a count is typically calculated as an average per cell. Thus, the AgNOR count gives an indication of generation time, a component of the rate of cellular proliferation. Higher AgNOR counts in MCTs are associated with increased mortality, local recurrence and metastasis. Lower AgNOR counts correlate with longer survival times but are not predictive of clinical behaviour independent of histological grade; this reduces the usefulness of the test since it does not provide prognostic information additional to that already provided by the Patnaik grade.

Ki67

Ki67 is a nuclear protein expressed in all active phases of the cell cycle, but which is not present in non-cycling cells. It is detected by immunohistochemical staining (Figure 7.3) and is calculated as the number of immunopositive cells per grid area, averaged over at least five grids OR by counting 1000 nuclei and expressing the relative proportion of positive nuclei as a percentage. Note that these two techniques are not interchangeable, and dif-

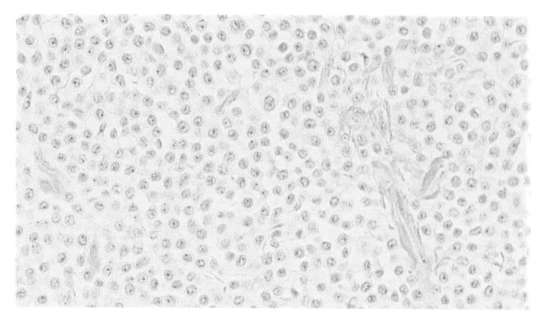

Figure 7.2 AgNOR staining of a canine MCT with a low count – count the dots!

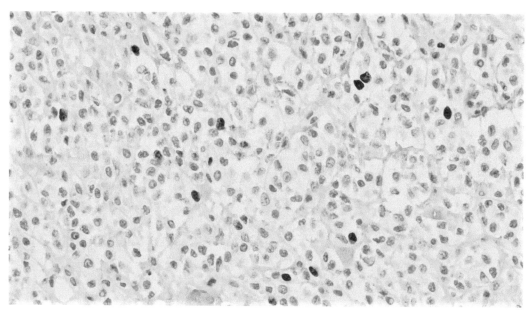

Figure 7.3 IHC staining for Ki67 on a canine MCT. Positive brown staining of nuclei, against a haematoxylin counterstain (pale blue).

ferent cut-off values are published for different techniques. The relative number of Ki67 positive cells indicates the growth fraction, or the relative number of cells actively involved in cell cycle growth at that point in time.

Studies have suggested that it is possible to divide Patnaik intermediate-grade (grade II) tumours into two groups based on the Ki67 score; those with higher Ki67 scores (Figure 7.4a) had shorter survival times than those with lower scores (Figure 7.4b). Ki67 has been shown to be a prognostic indicator independent

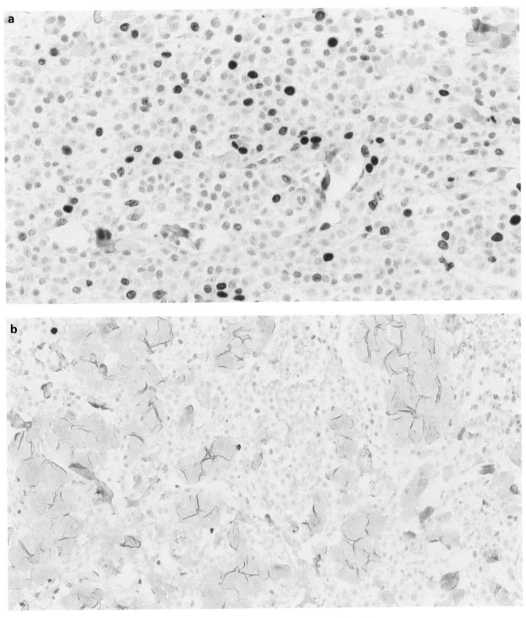

Figure 7.4 Ki67 IHC staining on a MCT with: (a) a high score; (b) a low score.

of histological grade, meaning it provides further prognostic information in addition to that given by the Patnaik grade. Interestingly one study reported that there was more grade I tumours with Ki67 scores above the reported cut-off level than there were grade II tumours. Of these high-scoring, grade I tumours, the majority were from dogs with multiple tumours, all of whom survived beyond the end of the study. This implies that the biological behaviour of tumours from dogs with multiple grade I masses is somehow different from the behaviour of solitary grade II tumours, and that Ki67 scores should still be interpreted in light of other relevant factors.

Combining Ki67 and AgNOR

The growth fraction (as measured by Ki67) is the proportion of cells within the tumour which are actively cycling, while the generation time (as measured by AgNOR) is the time taken by those cells to go through the cell cycle. Cellular proliferation is a product of both growth fraction and generation time, and so Ki67 and AgNOR scores are sometimes combined (also referred to as the Ag67 index) to give an indication of overall cellular proliferation within a tumour. Furthermore, the growth fraction and generation times are independent of one another, and thus are providing complementary biological information about the tumour cells, which may be more useful when the two indices are used in concert rather than individually.

c-KIT mutation

c-KIT is a proto-oncogene; these are normal genes that are involved in regulating cell growth and differentiation. c-KIT encodes a tyrosine kinase receptor (KIT), which is normally expressed on the cell surface and acts as a receptor for a growth factor called stem cell factor (Figure 7.5a). Mutations in the c-KIT gene convert it to an oncogene; these are genes that are abnormally activated and thus promote autonomous cell growth in cancer cells. Such mutations in the c-KIT gene can result in a KIT receptor which is permanently activated even in the absence of its stem cell factor ligand (Figure 7.5b). c-KIT mutations can be an important contributory factor in mast cell tumour development and growth, for example by increasing cellular proliferation (via both generation time and growth fraction). The percentage of tumours with a c-KIT mutation varies somewhat between studies, for example from 8.3% to 16%. There is an association between the presence of the mutation and a higher histological grade. c-KIT gene mutations are detectable by PCR, and although they are not necessarily always associated with a worse prognosis, knowledge of their presence may influence the choice of chemotherapeutic agents.

KIT staining patterns

KIT is the tyrosine kinase receptor encoded by the c-KIT gene, as discussed above. Normally, the KIT receptor is present on the cell surface (that is, membrane-associated), and several studies have looked for changes in KIT staining patterns in tumour cells and whether these are associated with outcome. Staining pattern I is membrane-associated staining with little or no cytoplasmic staining (that is, normal, Figure 7.6a), while staining pattern II is intense focal or stippled cytoplasmic staining (Figure 7.6b), and pattern III is diffuse cytoplasmic staining of neoplastic mast cells (Figure 7.6c). The overall pattern given is determined by the highest staining pattern present in at least 10% of the neoplastic cell population, or in large clusters of the neoplastic cells present. Staining patterns II and III, that is, increased cytoplasmic staining of KIT, are thought to be associated with shorter overall survival times and increased risk of local recurrence.

a

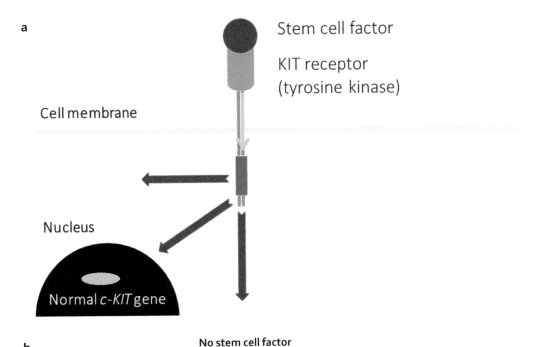

Stem cell factor

KIT receptor
(tyrosine kinase)

Cell membrane

Nucleus

Normal *c-KIT* gene

b

No stem cell factor

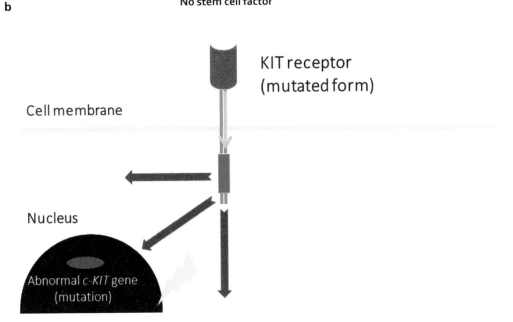

KIT receptor
(mutated form)

Cell membrane

Nucleus

Abnormal *c-KIT* gene
(mutation)

Figure 7.5 (a) Normal signalling pathway, with stem cell factor bound to the KIT receptor on the cell surface of the mast cell, stimulating appropriate activation of the receptor and intracellular signalling. (b) A mutation in the *c-KIT* gene has resulted in an abnormal KIT receptor protein, still expressed on the cell surface but now activated even in the absence of stem cell factor, promoting autonomous cell growth in this neoplastic mast cell.

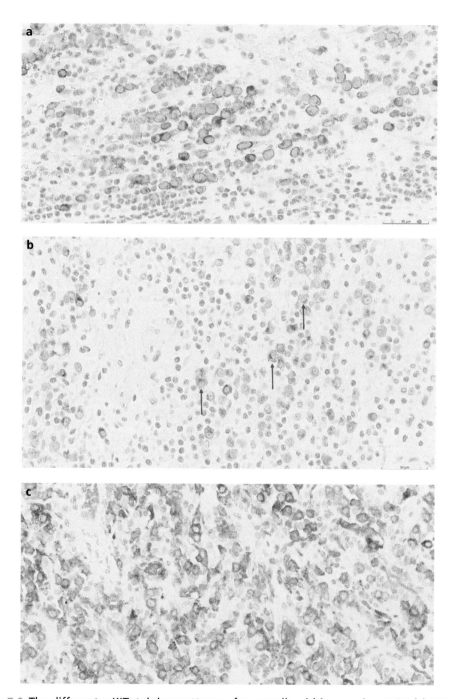

Figure 7.6 The different *c-KIT* staining patterns of mast cells within a canine MCT: (a) KIT staining pattern I, membrane-associated staining only; (b) KIT staining pattern II, loss of membrane-associated staining with focal or stippled cytoplasmic staining (red arrows); (c) KIT staining pattern III, diffuse cytoplasmic staining.

In some studies KIT staining pattern III was associated with Patnaik grade II and III tumours, while staining patterns I and II were associated with Patnaik grade I tumours. It is thought that the presence of KIT staining pattern I could be useful in predicting a good outcome (that is, low grade) in cases with a Patnaik grade II tumour. When data were analysed using the newly proposed two-tier histological grading system, one study found that most high-grade MCTs had staining pattern III, while low-grade tumours were mostly associated with staining patterns I and II – although this was not absolute. Studies also found that histological grade, *c-KIT* mutations and KIT staining patterns were all independent factors, thus all can theoretically provide useful prognostic information in their own right.

Subcutaneous MCTs

The vast majority of research into the use of these prognostic markers has been performed in cutaneous MCTs only. Initially, it was thought that markers such as AgNOR, Ki67 and KIT expression were not associated with prognosis in purely subcutaneous MCTs. However, more recently higher counts for Ki67, on its own or in combination with AgNOR, and cytoplasmic KIT staining patterns have been significantly associated with local recurrence and metastasis and therefore they may have some prognostic value for these tumours. Further work is needed looking at this subcutaneous variant, as well as MCTs arising at other sites.

Feline MCTs

Further prognostic tests which are routinely available for use in canine MCTs have been researched in feline cases, but most studies to date are still on the small side. One study looked at Ki67 and found that a higher score was correlated with an unfavourable outcome, but that it was also correlated with the mitotic count and so did not add much prognostic information for the clinician. This same study also looked at KIT staining patterns, dividing cases into the three patterns originally described and used for canine MCT prognostication and looking for aberrant KIT-protein expression. In terms of outcome (that is, dead or alive after 24 months), the 'alive' group had four cases with no KIT staining, seven cases with membranous (that is, normal) and seven cases with cytoplasmic (that is, aberrant), while the 'dead' group had five cases with cytoplasmic staining but none with either absent or membranous. A later study reported a correlation between cytoplasmic KIT staining and an unfavourable outcome, but it is unclear whether this adds any further useful prognostic information, since it was also correlated with an increased mitotic rate. This study also reported that mutations in the *c-KIT* gene (exons 8, 9 and 11) were present in 56% of tumours but were not significantly related to either the protein expression pattern or to the survival outcome. Interestingly, cats sometimes had multiple nodules which had different mutation statuses, suggesting that *c-KIT* mutations may play a rather complex role in the development of these multiple neoplasms.

Other studies have also looked at prognostication of feline MCTs, including KIT staining pattern and also another proliferation marker called MCM7. To date, the most useful prognostic feature is still the mitotic count. Studies have found a significant difference in survival times when comparing cats with tumours with a membranous KIT staining pattern (mean survival 1675 days) and cats with tumours with a cytoplasmic KIT staining pattern (mean survival 1177 days; figure 7.7). This finding is in agreement with those of the previous study (Sabattini et al., 2013), where cytoplasmic staining for KIT was associated with a poorer clinical outcome. Sabattini found that the relationship between the presence of *c-KIT* mutations, KIT staining patterns and clinical outcomes was complex in feline MCTs, and our study

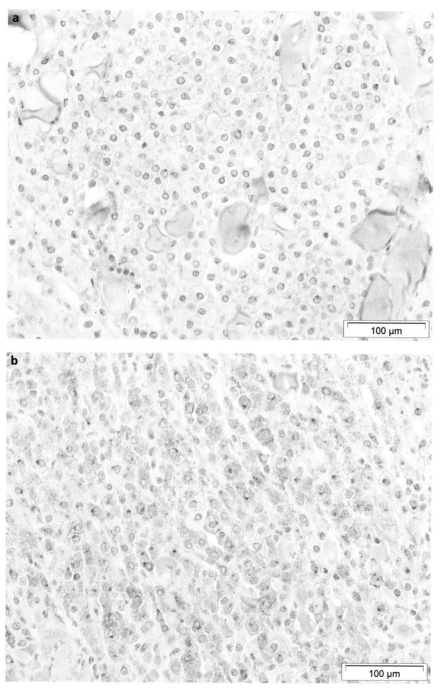

Figure 7.7 KIT IHC staining of a feline cutaneous MCT: (a) these mast cells demonstrate a membranous staining pattern for KIT; (b) these mast cells demonstrate a cytoplasmic staining pattern for KIT.

supported this. So, at this stage, there is insufficient evidence that this test is really particularly useful for prognostication.

Canine melanocytic neoplasms, oral and cutaneous

Table 7.7 usefully summarizes where we are with prognostication of these neoplasms. It is taken from the VCS/ACVP Oncology-Pathology Working Group Consensus on the Diagnosis of and Histopathologic Prognostication for Canine Melanocytic Neoplasms (Smedley et al., 2022), who adapted it from a paper published by Smedley et al. (2011).

Table 7.7 Current parameters for prognostication of canine melanocytic neoplasms, based on VCS/ACVP Oncology-Pathology Working Group Consensus (2022) and Smedley et al. (2011)

	Oral/lip melanocytic neoplasms	Cutaneous/digit melanocytic neoplasms
Distant metastasis	Poor prognosis	Poor prognosis
Lymphatic invasion	Poor prognosis	Poor prognosis[a]
Mitotic count[b]	<4/10 HPF = favourable prognosis	<3/10 HPF = favourable prognosis
	≥4/10 HPF = poor prognosis	≥3/10 HPF = poor prognosis
Nuclear atypia[c]	<30 = favourable prognosis	<20 = favourable prognosis
(% atypical nuclei)	≥30 = poor prognosis	≥20 = poor prognosis
Degree of pigmentation	% pigmented cells	Scale 0 (no pigment) to 2 (high pigment)
	≥50 = favourable prognosis	2 = favourable prognosis
	<50 = uncertain prognosis	0 to 1 = uncertain prognosis
Presence of ulceration	No prognostic significance	Poor prognosis
Level of infiltration/ invasion	Shallow or raised with no bone lysis = favourable prognosis	Limited to dermis = favourable prognosis
	Deep with possible bone lysis = poor prognosis	Extends beyond dermis = poor prognosis
Tumour thickness	Not investigated	≤0.95 cm tumour thickness[d] = favourable prognosis >0.95 cm tumour thickness[d] = poor prognosis
	Average number of positive nuclei per grid (5 HPF grid areas counted)	% of positive nuclei in 500 cells counted

Table 7.7 (continued)

	Oral/lip melanocytic neoplasms	Cutaneous/digit melanocytic neoplasms
Ki67 index	<19 = favourable prognosis	<15 = favourable prognosis
	≥19 = poor prognosis	≥15 = poor prognosis

Notes:

A favourable prognosis relates to expected survival times longer than one year and a poor prognosis relates to an expected death due to melanocytic neoplasia within less than one-year post-diagnosis for all melanocytic neoplasms. These predictions are based solely on publications that met the strict criteria for inclusion for each single parameter. These predictions do not take into account stage of disease or treatment strategies. When there are mixed results, results for each parameter should be reported, but Ki67 index should be used for final interpretation in most cases.

[a] Parameter was not specifically examined for neoplasms of the digit.

[b] For this consensus, the mitotic count (reported as mitotic index, in the literature reviewed) is obtained by counting the absolute number of mitoses in 10 high-power fields (400× magnification/40× objective or, ideally, in an area of 2.37 mm²) in the region with highest mitotic activity, as determined initially on a low power scan (100× magnification/10× objective) of the specimen.

[c] Parameter should be assessed in epithelioid predominant neoplasms and in spindloid neoplasms with sufficiently observable nuclear detail.

[d] Tumour thickness is measured with a ruler by placing the ruler on the glass slide perpendicular to the epidermis or mucosal epithelial surface and measuring the largest thickness of the tumour.

Some of these features can be assessed on the initial HE sections and may prompt the pathologist to suggest additional prognostic tests including Ki67 scoring. Note also that some of these features cannot be assessed on incisional biopsy samples and some are clinical (metastatic disease).

New markers and prognostic tests are being studied all the time, and I am sure with advanced technology including digital pathology, and image analysis, there will be rapid progress in this field. But we still clearly have some way to go and more work to do (Figure 7.8).

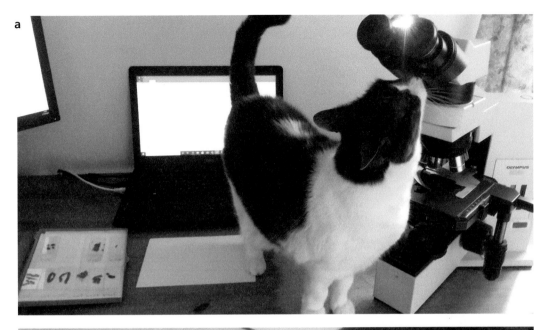

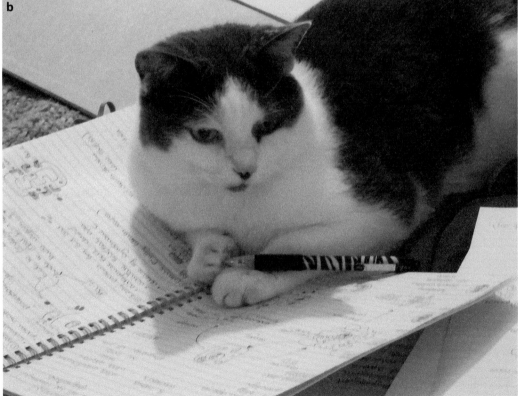

Figure 7.8 Clearly we still have a lot more work to do!

Self-assessment: 'What histological grade would you give?'

Part I – canine mast cell tumours

Case 1

One sample is received from a 4-year 6-month-old, female (neutered) Boxer. The clinical history is of a small mass on the right thorax/flank.

Key features The mass is confined to the dermis, is slightly raised and well-demarcated, with no evidence of ulceration or necrosis. The mass is composed of mast cells which are uniform in appearance with regular nuclei, and plenty of cytoplasmic granules. There are also some eosinophils present. There are no macro-, bi- or multi-nucleate cells present. The mitotic count is zero in 10 HPFs (400×; 2.37 mm^2).

1. What Patnaik and Kiupel grading would you assign to this MCT?
    Additional testing results:
    Ki67 = 10
    AgNOR = 2.2
    Ki67 × AgNOR (Ag67 index) = 22
    KIT pattern I
    Negative for *c-KIT* mutations (exon 7 and 11)
2. Are any of these results of cause for concern?

Case 2

One sample is received from a 12-year 11-month-old, female Golden retriever. The clinical history is of a cutaneous mass in the right axilla.

Key features The mass is located in the deep dermis and subcutis of the skin, composed of multifocal infiltrates which are not particularly well-demarcated from the surrounding tissues, and are associated with areas of haemorrhage as well as some degenerative changes. There are large numbers of eosinophils also present. The neoplastic cell population is round, with a variable degree of cytoplasmic granulation (a special Giemsa stain is needed to confirm the presence of cytoplasmic granules within the neoplastic round cell population). There is some variation in nuclear and cell size, with sometimes prominent nucleoli, and also some variation in nuclear shape. There are occasional bi-nucleate and macro-nucleate cells noted. The mitotic count is 13 in 10 HPFs (400×; 2.37 mm^2).

3. What Patnaik and Kiupel grading would you assign to this mast cell tumour?
    Additional testing results:
    Ki67 = 36.4
    AgNOR = 3.4
    KIAG = 123.76
    KIT pattern 2
    Negative for *c-KIT* mutations (exon 7 and 11)
4. Are any of these results of cause for concern?

Case 3

One sample is received from a 10-year 10-month-old, female Jack Russell terrier. The clinical history is of a cutaneous mass from the right lateral body wall.

Key features The mass is located within the dermis and superficial parts of the subcutis, and is moderately well-demarcated from the surrounding tissues. There is widespread ulceration of the surface. Most of the neoplastic cells are reasonably well-granulated and eosinophils are also present. There is moderate variation in nuclear and cell size, with sometimes prominent nucleoli, some variation in nuclear shape but no macro-, bi- or multi-nucleate mast cells seen. The mitotic count is 7 in 10 HPFs (400×; 2.37 mm²).

5. What Patnaik and Kiupel grading would you assign to this MCT?
   Additional testing results:
      Ki67 = 18
      AgNOR = 3.1
      KIAG = 55.8
      KIT pattern 2
      Negative for *c-KIT* mutations (exon 7 and 11)
6. Are any of these results of cause for concern?

Part II – canine soft tissue sarcoma (soft tissue tumours)

Case 4

This case is of an 8-year 9-month-old, male (neutered) crossbreed dog. Two masses are present, described as subcutaneous in location; the first is a lipoma but the second mass is a STS.

Key features The mass is well-demarcated from the surrounding tissues, but has a mildly infiltrative growth pattern. The tumour cells are well-differentiated and spindle-shaped, with mild anisocytosis. There is no evidence of necrosis within the mass, although there are some perivascular lymphoid aggregates present. There is mild anisokaryosis with sometimes prominent nucleoli but no bi- or multi-nucleate cells. The mitotic count is 3 in 10 HPFs (400×; 2.37 mm²).

7. What histological grade would you assign to this soft tissue sarcoma?

Case 5

This case is of a 9-year 7-month-old, male (neutered) Boxer. The clinical history is of a large mass on the cranial aspect of the left stifle. The mass is described as having tripled in size in 6 weeks.

Key features The mass is moderately well-demarcated from the surrounding tissues, but has a peripherally infiltrative growth pattern and varies in cellularity depending on the field examined. The tumour cells are well-differentiated and spindle-shaped, elongated to polygonal in shape, with small to moderate amounts of cytoplasm and moderate anisocytosis. There are some small focal areas of necrosis within the mass, and extensive inflammatory cell infiltrates. There is moderate anisokaryosis with sometimes prominent nucleoli. The mitotic count is 10 in 10 HPFs (400×; 2.37 mm²).

8. What histological grade would you assign to this soft tissue sarcoma?

Case 6

This case is of an 8-year 3-month-old, male (neutered) Springer spaniel dog. The clinical history is of a mass on the caudal aspect of the right hind limb.

Key features This mass is moderately cellular, unencapsulated, infiltrative and moderately well-demarcated from the surrounding tissues, and contains multifocal, often extensive areas of necrosis accounting for more than 50% of the tumour present in these sections. There is moderate anisocytosis, and moderate to marked anisokaryosis, with some multi-nucleate cells and a mitotic count of 32 in 10 HPFs (400×; 2.37 mm²).

9. What histological grade would you assign to this soft tissue sarcoma?

The answers are available on page 185.

Self-assessment answers

Chapter 1

Self-assessment: multiple choice questions

1 A GREAT DANE HAS UNDERGONE LIMB AMPUTATION SURGERY FOR A SUSPECTED BONE TUMOUR AFFECTING THE DISTAL FEMUR. YOU WANT TO SUBMIT THE SAMPLE FOR HISTOLOGICAL ASSESSMENT, BUT IS FAR TOO LARGE FOR ANY OF THE ROUTINE SAMPLE POTS. WHICH OF THE FOLLOWING SHOULD YOU DO?

   a Wrap the sample in formalin-soaked gauze to keep it moist in transit and submit it straight away before it undergoes autolysis.

   b Ensure all of the skin, muscle, lymph nodes and marginal tissues are kept together, as it is vital that all of it is submitted for assessment in one piece.

   c Remove normal tissues like muscle and skin, cut down the sample to the portion of bone with the lesion and place in fixative as soon as possible.

   d Ensure there is a 5:1 formalin:tissue ratio so that the sample will fix nice and slowly.

   (c) Remove normal tissues like muscle and skin, cut down the sample to the portion of bone with the lesion and place in fixative as soon as possible.

   Debulking normal tissues that do not need to be assessed means that the remaining essential tissues fix faster and the tissue detail will be better preserved, as the formalin has less tissue to penetrate through before reaching the critical lesion. This also means less volume of formalin is required to fix the sample and a smaller sample for transportation to the laboratory.

2 SAMPLE CONTAINERS SHOULD BE:

   a easily breakable so that the sample can be retrieved by the laboratory personnel

   b screw-top, water-tight and designed for the purpose of submitting samples for histopathology

   c re-enforced with surgical or duct tape in case of formalin leakage during transit

   d small enough that the sample will be held snugly in place during transit, to avoid damaging the sample.

   (b) screw-top, water-tight and designed for the purpose of submitting samples for histopathology

   Sample containers should be non-breakable, and should not need to be re-enforced with surgical or duct tape to make them water-tight.

3 WHAT DETAILS DO NOT NEED TO BE ON A SAMPLE SUBMISSION FORM?
   a The animal's age.
   b The practice details.
   c The owner's phone number.
   d Where the sample was taken from.
      (c) The owner's phone number.
           The laboratory and the pathologist need details about the lesion, the animal and the prac-
           tice, but not the owner (other than surname for purposes of identifying the patient).

4 YOU SHOULD NEVER PACKAGE CYTOLOGY AND HISTOPATHOLOGY SAMPLES TOGETHER BECAUSE:
   a the laboratory might get them muddled up and perform the wrong test on the wrong sample
   b if one sample gets lost in transit, you should still have the second sample
   c the formalin fumes will make the labels come off
   d the formalin fumes will affect the cytology samples.
      (d) the formalin fumes will affect the cytology samples
           Formalin fumes will cause severe artefact in the cytology samples and render them largely
           uninterpretable.

5 CRUSH ARTEFACT CAN RESULT IN WHAT CHANGES IN THE TISSUES:
   a nuclear streaming, with loss of nuclear detail
   b the tissue to swell in size and become less malleable
   c damage of the tissues due to heat
   d loss of the mucosal layer.
      (a) nuclear streaming, with loss of nuclear detail
           Particularly in some tissues with fragile cells, for example neoplastic cells or lymphoid
           tissues. Nuclear streaming results in loss of nuclear detail, including nuclear morphology,
           whether the cell population is mixed, the degree of anisokaryosis (variation in nuclear size)
           and whether there is any evidence of mitotic activity.

Self-assessment: case study

Case background

The patient is a 10-year-old, female (neutered) domestic short hair cat named Poppy, belonging to a Mr
and Mrs Doolittle. Poppy initially presented to you a fortnight ago, when she had a palpable but rather
indistinct, subcutaneous swelling over the inner aspect of the upper left forelimb. Today the physical
examination suggests it is extending to involve the ventral thorax on that side. The area is dark pink
to red and warm to the touch, and she rather resents you palpating it. The axillary and pre-scapular
lymph nodes feel slightly enlarged on the left side when compared to the right. Physical examination
does not reveal any other lymphadenopathy or lesions, and she is not pyrexic or otherwise systemically
unwell. She has now been treated with antibiotics for 2 weeks without any obvious sign of improvement. A previous cytology sample came back as inflammatory, but with no evidence of infectious
agents. You decide further investigation is warranted and that you wish to submit further samples to the
laboratory.

Please answer the following questions.

1 WHAT ARE YOUR DIFFERENTIAL DIAGNOSES?
- Neoplastic, with metastatic spread to the regional lymph nodes.
- Inflammatory/infectious, with reactive hyperplasia of the lymph nodes.
- Migrating foreign body, penetrating injury, foreign material implantation, trauma.

2 WHAT SAMPLES WOULD YOU SUBMIT AND HOW WOULD YOU PRESERVE THESE?
- FNA of the enlarged lymph node – prepare slides in-house, check for suitability, and make sure to submit cytology samples separate from any histology samples (due to the effects of formalin fumes).
- Biopsy of the mass or swelling; some tissue should be placed in formalin for histological assessment..
- Fresh tissue (i.e. not fixed) for microbial culture (you could either submit at the same time, or keep in the fridge in the practice pending the histology results).

3 WHAT CONTACT INFORMATION NEEDS TO BE INCLUDED ON THE FORM?
Your practice details, the submitting veterinary surgeon's name, the preferred method of receiving the report if this is not already set up with the laboratory (make sure details such as email addresses are up-to-date).

4 WHAT INFORMATION IS REQUIRED ABOUT THE OWNER AND ANIMAL?
"Poppy" Doolittle; 10 years old, female (neutered) Domestic short hair cat.

5 CAN YOU PROVE A CLINICAL SUMMARY – MAXIMUM 200 WORDS?
Subcutaneous, dark pink to red, warm and possibly painful swelling, two weeks duration, affecting the inner left forelimb and now extending to the ventral thorax. Possible enlargement of local lymph nodes. Non-responsive to antibiosis, previous cytology results suggestive of inflammatory process, but with no evidence of infectious agents.
Type of samples submitted and site(s) taken from …

6 IS THERE ANY OTHER EXTRA INFORMATION YOU WOULD LIKE TO INCLUDE?
Suggestions:
- The type of antibiotics tried and that they appeared not to work
- Any other therapy tried
- Any imaging performed
- Any previous history which may potentially be relevant – history of trauma, other masses etc.
- Any systemic signs or lack of, such as pyrexia.
- Any other test results which may be relevant.
- Photographs

Chapter 2

Self-assessment: gross lesion descriptions

Have a try at a gross description for each lesion shown in Figure 2.14. Remember to think about the number, shape, colour, demarcation and the lesion distribution.

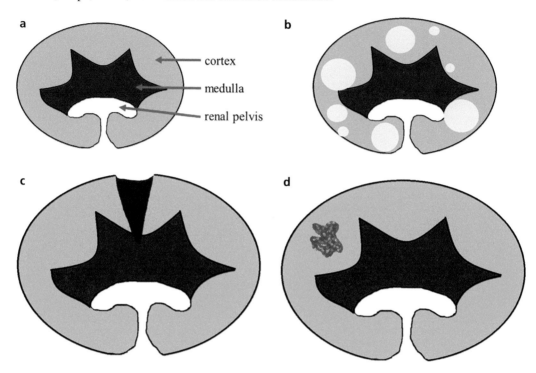

Figure 2.14a–d (a) A schematic diagram of a kidney, with the cortex, medulla and renal pelvis labelled. (b–d) Images of different lesions arising in the kidney.

Gross description answers

(b) Multifocal (8), variably sized, well-demarcated, spherical, pale yellow lesions with a smooth edge; present scattered randomly within the renal cortex and rarely impinging on the medulla.

(c) A single, well-demarcated, dark brown and wedge-shaped or triangular lesion, extending from a focal point in the medulla and radiating outwards through the cortex to the surface, which is indented.

(d) A single, irregular-shaped, moderately well-demarcated, mottled pink to red lesion within the cortex.

Self-assessment: quick quiz

1 WHAT ARE THE MAIN ORGANS AND STRUCTURES WHICH MAKE UP THE 'PLUCK'?

Lungs, tongue, oropharynx, larynx, trachea, heart, oesophagus, mediastinum, thymus in young animals

2 WHAT DOES IT MEAN IF A PORTION OF LUNG TISSUE FLOATS IN FORMALIN?

It suggests the lung tissue contains air, that is, it is aerated, rather than containing anything more solid.

3 HOW WOULD YOU CHECK FOR THE PRESENCE OF NEGATIVE PRESSURE IN THE THORACIC CAVITY?

Having opened the abdominal cavity, watch closely as you make a small stab incision through the diaphragm; in the presence of negative pressure in the thoracic cavity there should be an influx of air into the thorax as you make the incision. You should see the diaphragm 'relax' and move slightly towards the abdominal cavity, and you might hear the influx of air also.

4 WHAT IS THE NORMAL RATIO OF THICKNESS OF THE RIGHT VENTRICULAR FREE WALL (RVFW), INTERVENTRICULAR SEPTUM AND LEFT VENTRICULAR FREE WALL (LVFW)?

In a normal healthy animal, the expected ratio of the RVFW, interventricular septum and LVFW would be 1 : 3 : 3. So for example, in a feline heart, the RVFW might measure 1 mm, the interventricular septum 3 mm and the LVFW 3 mm. This should be measured perpendicular to the long axis at approximately one-third of the way up from the apex, avoiding the papillary muscles.

5 HOW WOULD YOU CHECK FOR PATENCY OF THE BILE DUCT?

Having opened the abdominal cavity, and located the gall bladder and duodenum, first make a small incision into the duodenum so you can visualize the mucosa. Apply gentle pressure to the gall bladder and watch to see if bile is observed entering the duodenum.

Chapter 3

Self-assessment: multiple choice questions

1 IN WHICH OF THE FOLLOWING TYPES OF MARGIN ASSESSMENT CAN THE LATERAL AND DEEP MARGINS BE MEASURED?

a Tumour bed technique
b Cross-sectional
c Tangential
d Shaved

    (b) Cross-sectional. All of the other forms of margin assessment give a binary result, either positive or negative for the presence of neoplastic cells, and cannot provide a measurement.

2 WHAT IS THE HISTOLOGICAL TUMOUR FREE MARGIN?

   a The distance between the mass and the surgical margin as seen grossly at the time of surgery.
   b The distance between the neoplastic tissue and the margin as seen microscopically.
   c The degree of tumour invasiveness.
   d The distance between the mass and the surgical margin as seen grossly by the pathologist once the sample is completely fixed.

      (b) The distance between the neoplastic tissue and the margin as seen microscopically.

3 WHAT IS THE RELATIONSHIP BETWEEN THE GROSS MARGIN YOU SEE SURGICALLY AND THE DISTANCE MEASURED ON THE SLIDE BY THE PATHOLOGIST?

   a They are the same in size.
   b The gross margin is smaller than the distance measured on the slide.
   c The gross margin is larger than the distance measured on the slide by a factor of at least 10.
   d The gross margin is larger than the distance measured on the slide but the factor varies.

      (d) The gross margin is larger than the distance measured on the slide but the factor varies. Tissue shrinks at various stages in the process, including surgical retraction once the tissue is removed from the patient, as well as during fixation and processing. The degree by which it shrinks is not predictable however, and varies between different tissue types.

4 WHAT TYPE OF MARGIN ASSESSMENT THEORETICALLY ALLOWS COMPLETE ASSESSMENT OF ALL MARGINAL TISSUES?

   a Cross-sectional
   b Bread loafing
   c Tangential
   d Pie

      (c) Tangential (also known as shaved margins).

5 USING SUTURE TAGS TO INDICATE AREAS OF INTEREST IS A GOOD IDEA, BUT YOU MUST:

   a make sure you bed them in nice and tight, so they do not fall off in transit
   b make sure they are all the same colour
   c remember to include what type of suture material you have used
   d none of the above.

      (d) none of the above. Using suture tags is a great way of indicating areas of interest or concern, but we must be able to remove then before sectioning, and we must be able to tell them apart if you indicate more than one site!

Self-assessment: case study

The patient is a 9-year-old, male (neutered) Golden retriever dog, who has presented with a mass on the distal left forelimb. The client says the mass has suddenly appeared in the last week, is increasing in size quickly and that the dog is self-traumatizing it. On a fine needle aspirate you diagnose the mass as a mast cell tumour. Palpation of the left pre-scapular lymph node reveals it is slightly larger than the right pre-scapular lymph node, so you obtain a further fine needle aspirate from the right pre-scapular lymph node for submission to the laboratory, and plan to perform a surgical excision of the mass. The anatomical location is difficult, as you feel margins will be difficult to achieve.

- WHEN SUBMITTING THE FINE NEEDLE ASPIRATE SAMPLE FROM THE RIGHT PRE-SCAPULAR LYMPH NODE FOR CYTOLOGICAL ASSESSMENT, HOW SHOULD YOU PACKAGE THIS (THINK BACK TO CHAPTER 1)?

  The key point is to ensure you package any cytology samples separately from the formalin-fixed specimen, as the formalin fumes will cause severe artefact and make the cytology sample potentially non-diagnostic.

- THE SURGICALLY EXCISED MASS IS TOO LARGE FOR A ROUTINE SAMPLE POT, WHAT SHOULD YOU DO (THINK BACK TO CHAPTER 1)?

  There are several possible solutions.
  - You could divide the sample into half or quarters if they then fit into the specimen pots, making sure you clearly label the pots and draw a diagram to illustrate how you have divided the mass.
  - Or, you could fix the mass first in the practice for a day or two, refreshing the formalin if needs be after 24 hours. Once the mass is fully fixed, wrap it in formalin-soaked gauze, place inside two sealed leak-proof bags, wrap in absorbent material and place inside a rigid container.
  - Or, you could submit tissue slices, remembering to include parts of the mass itself, the junction between the mass and adjacent tissues and the areas of most concern regards the margins. Retain the remainder of the fixed tissue sample at the practice while awaiting the report.

- YOU ARE PARTICULARLY WORRIED ABOUT THE DEEP MARGINS, AND ONE OF THE LATERAL MARGINS; WHAT CAN YOU DO TO HELP THE PATHOLOGIST ACCURATELY ASSESS THOSE PARTICULAR MARGINS?

  There are several possible solutions.
  - You could use suture tags to indicate the areas you are most concerned about, so that the laboratory staff know to assess those areas in particular – remember to clearly indicate on the submission form what the tags are highlighting.
  - You could apply tissue ink to either the whole of the surgical margin, or to the areas of most concern. Again, remember to include this information on the submission form.
  - You could sample additional tissues from the tumour bed at these sites of concern, and submit them separately to the main sample for assessment for the presence or absence of tumour cells – remember again to include this information on the submission form.

Chapter 4

Self-assessment: multiple choice questions

An 11-year-old, female (neutered) domestic short hair cat with a long history of intermittent vomiting and inappetence has now presented to your clinic with diarrhoea and progressive weight loss. The owner agrees to GI endoscopy and biopsy as part of investigation.

1 WHEN SUBMITTING THE ENDOSCOPIC GI BIOPSIES:
   a you should include a clinical history and signalment, including the symptoms, their duration and any previous and/or current treatments and any clinical response to those treatments
   b place samples from each level of the GI tract in a cell-safe, and then into an individual, labelled sample pot
   c remember that only the mucosa will be available for assessment by the pathologist and this may limit what information can be gained from the biopsies
   d all of the above are true.
      (d) all of the above!

2 SAMPLES FROM THE SMALL INTESTINES SHOW A DIFFUSE INFILTRATE PREDOMINANTLY COMPOSED OF SMALL LYMPHOCYTES. WHAT FEATURES PRESENT ON THE HE SECTIONS MIGHT RAISE CONCERN FOR A LOW-GRADE ALIMENTARY LYMPHOMA?
   a plasma cells admixed with the lymphocytes
   b villi which are equal in width and length, with no evidence of villous blunting or fusion
   c increased numbers of intra-epithelial lymphocytes which obscure the interface between the epithelial layer and the lamina propria
   d infiltrates confined to the mucosal layer
      (c) increased numbers of intra-epithelial lymphocytes which obscure the interface between the epithelial layer and the lamina propria – particularly if they form nests or plaques.

3 WHAT ADDITIONAL TESTING MIGHT YOU CONSIDER TO CONFIRM OR EXCLUDE THE POTENTIAL DIFFERENTIAL DIAGNOSIS OF LOW-GRADE ALIMENTARY LYMPHOMA? (THERE IS MORE THAN ONE CORRECT ANSWER HERE!)
   a immunohistochemical (IHC) staining for B-lymphocytes and T-lymphocytes
   b PARR testing for clonality, no need for IHC
   c immunohistochemical staining for B-lymphocytes and T-lymphocytes, followed by PARR testing if the infiltrate is predominantly T-cell on IHC and further confirmation is wanted
   d special staining for bacteria
      (a) immunohistochemical (IHC) staining for B-lymphocytes and T-lymphocytes
      OR
      (c) immunohistochemical staining for B-lymphocytes and T-lymphocytes, followed by PARR testing if the infiltrate is predominantly T-cell on IHC and further confirmation is wanted

4 WHICH OF THE FOLLOWING STRUCTURES ARE NOT PRESENT IN PORTAL TRACTS OF THE LIVER?
   a biliary ducts
   b hepatocytes
   c portal venules
   d hepatic arterioles
       (b) hepatocytes

5 HOW MANY COMPLETE PORTAL TRACTS ARE REQUIRED TO ADEQUATELY ASSESS THE LIVER FOR DIFFUSE CONDI-
   TIONS IN HUMAN MEDICINE?
   a 11–15
   b 1–5
   c 25
   d 50
       (a) 11–15

6 WHICH OF THE FOLLOWING SPECIAL STAINS IS USED TO DETECT THE PRESENCE OF COPPER IN LIVER BIOPSIES?
   a Perls
   b Masson's trichrome
   c Fouchet
   d Rhodanine
       (d) Rhodanine

7 THE PRESENCE OF WHICH OF THE FOLLOWING FEATURES IN LIVER BIOPSIES FROM A DOG WOULD SUGGEST A
   SECONDARY OR REACTIVE HEPATOPATHY RATHER THAN A PRIMARY INFLAMMATORY HEPATOPATHY?
   a hepatocyte necrosis
   b fibrosis
   c inflammatory cells in sinusoids
   d hepatocyte apoptosis
       (c) inflammatory cells in sinusoids

Chapter 5

Self-assessment: 'What's your diagnosis?'

Case 1

A 9-year 6-month-old female (neutered) domestic short hair cat presents with an intestinal mass, which is surgically resected and submitted for histopathology.

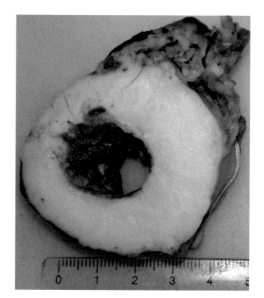

Figure 5.32a Appearance on gross assessment of the formalin-fixed specimen. The full circumference of the intestine is expanded by a soft, homogenous cream mass, with loss of the normal layering.

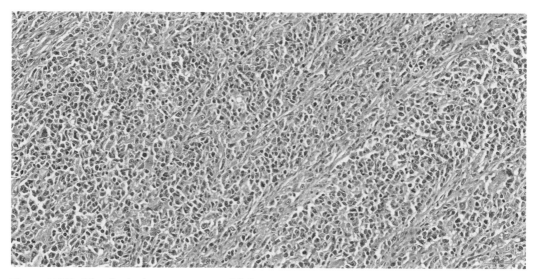

Figure 5.32b Histological appearance, at high power, stained with HE. The diagnosis is of an intestinal lymphoma, diffuse, large cell, with a high mitotic count. Immunohistochemical staining is performed.

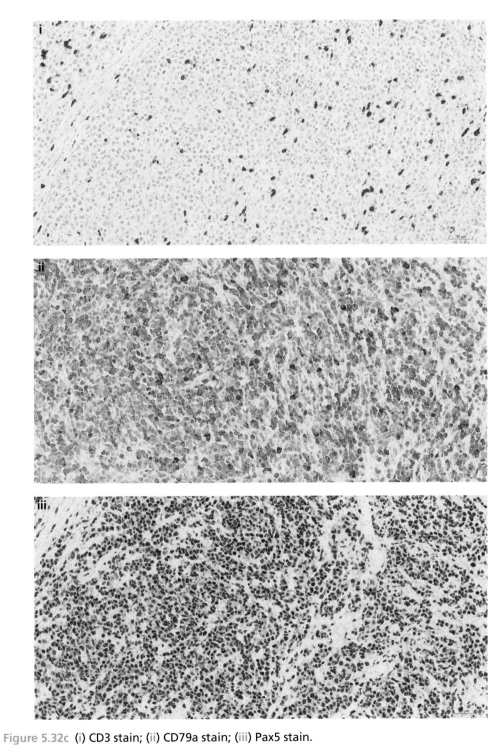

Figure 5.32c (i) CD3 stain; (ii) CD79a stain; (iii) Pax5 stain.

FIGURE 5.32C SHOWS THE RESULTS OF THE IMMUNOHISTOCHEMICAL STAINS FOR T-LYMPHOCYTES AND B-LYMPHOCYTES. WHAT IMMUNOPHENOTYPE DO YOU THINK THIS LYMPHOMA IS, T-CELL OR B-CELL?

The neoplastic cell population demonstrates positive staining for the two B-cell markers CD79a (cytoplasmic) and Pax5 (nuclear), and is negative staining for T-cell marker CD3 (there are a small number of positive-staining reactive T-cells which are not neoplastic). This is consistent with a B-cell lymphoma.

Case 2

A 4-year-old male (neutered) domestic long hair cat has had a submandibular swelling for 2 months. He has access to outdoors, is fully vaccinated and a known hunter of small rodents. He is systemically well and has no other lesions on physical examination. The swelling has not responded to a 2 week course of broad spectrum antibiotic medication. A biopsy is taken for histopathological assessment (Figure 5.33a).

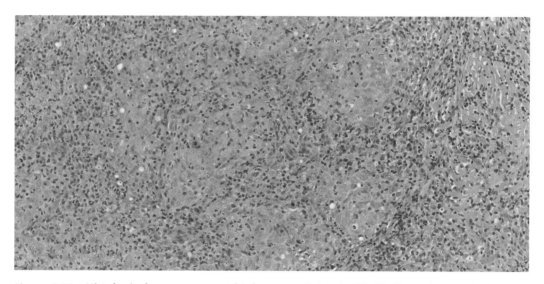

Figure 5.33a Histological appearance, at high power, stained with HE. There is a marked, diffuse and locally extensive, mixed inflammatory cell infiltrate present, which includes clusters and aggregates of reactive macrophages together with variable numbers of neutrophils, some lymphocytes and plasma cells.

1 BASED ON THIS INITIAL ASSESSMENT, WHAT ARE YOUR DIFFERENTIAL DIAGNOSES?

This is a granulomatous to pyogranulomatous inflammatory process.

Possible differential diagnoses include various types of infectious agent, such as bacteria including Mycobacteria, fungi, some viral infections (like FIP), protozoa.

Other possible causes might include a foreign body reaction, or a sterile granulomatous inflammatory process, xanthoma.

2 WHAT ADDITIONAL SPECIAL STAINS MIGHT YOU REQUEST AND WHY?

Special stains for infectious agents including Gram (bacteria), Ziehl–Neelsen (acid-fast bacteria, that is, Mycobacteria), PAS/Grocotts for fungi.

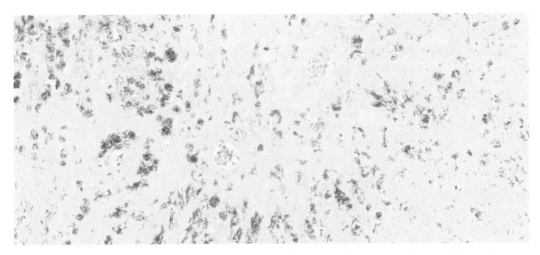

Figure 5.33b Can you identify this special stain, and is it positive or negative in this case?

3 LOOKING AT FIGURE 5.33B, CAN YOU IDENTIFY THIS SPECIAL STAIN, AND IS IT POSITIVE OR NEGATIVE IN THIS CASE?

This is a Ziehl–Neelsen stain; the positive-staining organisms are dark red and are present in very large numbers in this case!

Case 3

A 10-year-old male (neutered) Maine coon cat presents to your clinic with a history of acute collapse, which is found to be due to a haemoabdomen. On exploratory laparotomy, a ruptured splenic mass is discovered and a splenectomy performed. Representative sections are submitted for histopathology (Figure 5.34a).

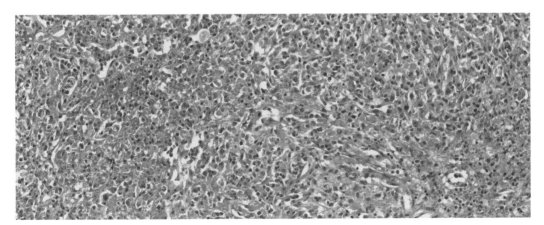

Figure 5.34a HE stained section showing parts of an unencapsulated, infiltrative neoplastic mass associated with extensive areas of necrosis and haemorrhage. The appearance is most consistent with a sarcoma. In some fields, there appears to be formation of vascular spaces lined by the neoplastic cells, but elsewhere the growth pattern is more solid.

1 WHAT TYPES OF SARCOMA CAN ARISE IN THE SPLEEN OF BOTH DOGS AND CATS, AND WHICH IS OF MOST CONCERN IN THIS CASE?

Smooth muscle origin (leiomyosarcoma), fibroblast origin (fibrosarcoma), endothelial cell origin (haemangiosarcoma), other forms are rare in cats (for example, histiocytic sarcoma, stromal sarcoma). You could also consider a metastatic lesion in this case, arising from a primary tumour elsewhere.

2 WHAT IMMUNOHISTOCHEMICAL STAINS MIGHT BE SUGGESTED IN THIS CASE?

Vimentin to confirm mesenchymal origin, smooth muscle actin for leiomyosarcoma, CD31 / Factor VIII for haemangiosarcoma, possibly histiocytic markers for histiocytic sarcoma.

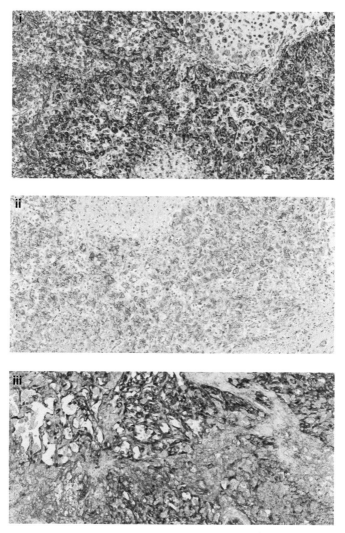

Figure 5.34b Immunohistochemical staining: (i) vimentin ; (ii) CD31; (iii) factor VIII (von Willebrand's factor).

Immunohistochemical staining is performed (Figure 5.34b) with the following:

a VIMENTIN – IS THE NEOPLASTIC CELL POPULATION POSITIVE OR NEGATIVE STAINING? WHAT DOES THIS TELL US?

The neoplastic cell population demonstrates positive staining for vimentin, confirming this is a tumour of mesenchymal cell origin, that is, a sarcoma.

b CD31 AND FACTOR VIII (VON WILLEBRAND'S FACTOR) – IS THE NEOPLASTIC CELL POPULATION POSITIVE OR NEGATIVE STAINING? WHAT DOES THIS TELL US?

The neoplastic cell population demonstrates positive staining for both of these markers for endothelial cells. This is supportive of a diagnosis of a haemangiosarcoma in this cat's spleen, particularly when taken in conjunction with the appearance of the HE stained sections.

c WHAT IS YOUR FINAL DIAGNOSIS IN THIS CASE?

Splenic haemangiosarcoma – presumed to be the primary tumour, but further staging and assessment strongly advisable.

Case 4

A 5-month-old male domestic long hair kitten presents with an area of scabbing and crusting under the left nostril (Figure 5.35a), but no obvious nasal or ocular discharge, no other lesions on the skin or evidence of fleas. The owner reports that a sibling has a similar facial lesion.

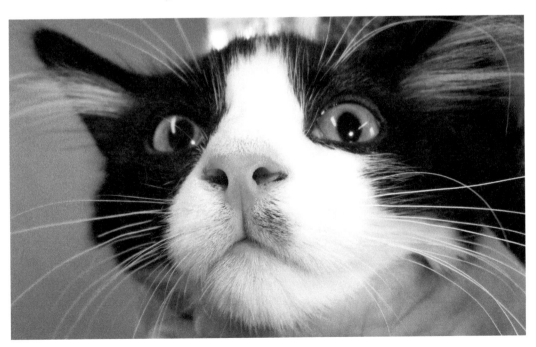

Figure 5.35a Photograph of the lesion.

1 SKIN BIOPSIES ARE SUBMITTED FOR HISTOPATHOLOGY. WHAT MIGHT YOUR LIST OF POSSIBLE DIFFERENTIAL DIAGNOSES INCLUDE AT THIS STAGE?

The list might be quite long! Hypersensitivity – eosinophilic granuloma complex; food hypersensitivity; Infectious agents – feline herpesvirus, calicivirus, pox virus, bacterial infection, fungal infection ('ringworm'), ectoparasites; trauma / self-trauma.

Figure 5.35b shows a HE stained section at lower power, through haired skin and the keratin layer. It shows hyperplasia of the epidermis (acanthosis) and also hyperkeratosis. There is a mild, perivascular to interstitial, mixed dermatitis.

2 CAN YOU IDENTIFY THE OBJECTS WITHIN THE KERATIN LAYER, HIGHLIGHTED BY THE RED ARROWS?

There are lightly basophilic, round to ovoid bodies, some of which are budding ('boot-prints'). These are suggestive of a yeast-like organism, such as Malassezia.

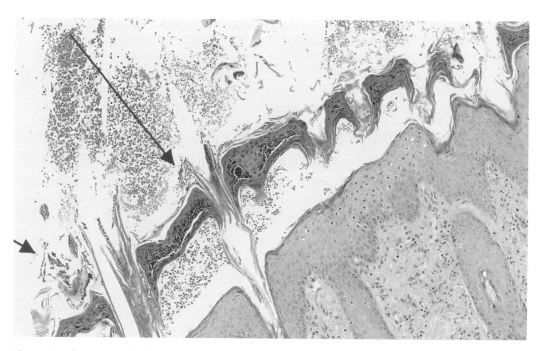

Figure 5.35b A HE stained section at lower power.

Figure 5.35c shows a higher power view of the HE stained section.

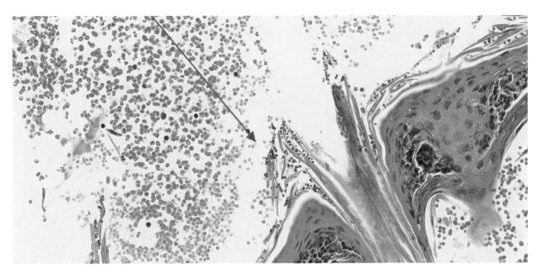

Figure 5.35c A higher power view of the HE stained section.

3 WHAT SPECIAL STAINS WHICH YOU SUGGEST IN THIS CASE?

You might suggest special stains for fungi, such as PAS or Grocotts, and you might also suggest Gram to look for any bacterial organisms also. It is unusual to see Malassezia in feline skin biopsies; although superficial yeast infection (like superficial staphylococcal infection) can be primary, it can also be seen secondary to other skin disorders. As the sibling also has similar lesions, it may be worth screening for any possible underlying causes which may have predisposed to this infection.

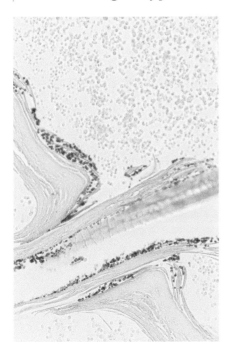

Figure 5.35d Can you identify this stain?

4 CAN YOU IDENTIFY THIS STAIN IN FIGURE 5.35D?

Grocott's methenamine silver stain. The fungal organisms are dark brown to black.

Chapter 6

Self-assessment: quick fire quiz

1 WHICH OF THE FOLLOWING NEOPLASMS IS CONSIDERED BENIGN?
   a Hepatocellular carcinoma
   b Liposarcoma
   c Haemangioma
   d Rhabdomyosarcoma
      (c) Haemangioma

2 WHICH OF THE FOLLOWING CHARACTERISTICS IS CONSIDERED THE DEFINITIVE CRITERION FOR MALIGNANCY?
   a Frequent metastasis
   b Capsule often present
   c Normal appearing mitotic figures
   d Well-differentiated appearance
      (a) Frequent metastasis

3 WHICH OF THE FOLLOWING IS INCORRECT?
   a Neoplasm means 'new growth'
   b Cancer means 'crab'
   c Metastasis means 'change of place'
   d Tumour means 'neoplastic'
      (d) Tumour means 'neoplastic' (tumour means 'swelling')

4 WHICH OF THE FOLLOWING CAN BE CONSIDERED A HALLMARK OF DIFFERENTIATION?
   a Loss of normal tissue architecture
   b Hypertrophy
   c Inflammation
   d The presence of portal tracts
      (a) Loss of normal tissue architecture

5 WHICH OF THE FOLLOWING IS A CELLULAR FEATURE?
   a Anisokaryosis
   b Multinucleation
   c Abnormal mitotic figures
   d Anisocytosis
      (d) Anisocytosis (all of the others are nuclear features)

Chapter 7

Self-assessment: 'What histological grade would you give?'

Part I – canine mast cell tumours

CASE 1

One sample is received from a 4-year 6-month-old, female (neutered) Boxer. The clinical history is of a small mass on the right thorax/flank.

Key features The mass is confined to the dermis, is slightly raised and well-demarcated, with no evidence of ulceration or necrosis. The mass is composed of mast cells which are uniform in appearance with regular nuclei, and plenty of cytoplasmic granules. There are also some eosinophils present. There are no macro-, bi- or multi-nucleate cells present. The mitotic count is zero in 10 HPFs (400×; 2.37 mm²).

  1 WHAT PATNAIK AND KIUPEL GRADING WOULD YOU ASSIGN TO THIS MCT?
    This mass is a Patnaik low grade (grade I) and Kiupel low grade.

Additional testing results:
  Ki67 = 10
  AgNOR = 2.2
  Ki67 × AgNOR (Ag67 index) = 22
  KIT pattern I
  Negative for *c-KIT* mutations (exon 7 and 11)

  2 ARE ANY OF THESE RESULTS OF CAUSE FOR CONCERN?
    No, they are all below the threshold values.

CASE 2

One sample is received from a 12-year 11-month-old, female Golden retriever. The clinical history is of a cutaneous mass in the right axilla.

Key features The mass is located in the deep dermis and subcutis of the skin, composed of multifocal infiltrates which are not particularly well-demarcated from the surrounding tissues, and are associated with areas of haemorrhage as well as some degenerative changes. There are large numbers of eosinophils also present. The neoplastic cell population is round, with a variable degree of cytoplasmic granulation (a special Giemsa stain is needed to confirm the presence of cytoplasmic granules within the neoplastic round cell population). There is some variation in nuclear and cell size, with sometimes prominent nucleoli, and also some variation in nuclear shape. There are occasional bi-nucleate and macro-nucleate cells noted. The mitotic count is 13 in 10 HPFs (400×; 2.37 mm²).

  3 WHAT PATNAIK AND KIUPEL GRADING WOULD YOU ASSIGN TO THIS MAST CELL TUMOUR?
    This mass is a Patnaik high grade (grade III) and of Kiupel high grade.

Additional testing results:
   Ki67 = 36.4
   AgNOR = 3.4
   KIAG = 123.76
   KIT pattern 2
   Negative for *c-KIT* mutations (exon 7 and 11)

   4   ARE ANY OF THESE RESULTS OF CAUSE FOR CONCERN?
       Ki67 (cut-off value is 23), KIAG (cut-off value is 54). KIT pattern II possibly of cause for concern,
       depending on the study you read!

CASE 3

One sample is received from a 10-year 10-month-old, female Jack Russell terrier. The clinical history is of
a cutaneous mass from the right lateral body wall.

Key features The mass is located within the dermis and superficial parts of the subcutis, and is moderately well-demarcated from the surrounding tissues. There is widespread ulceration of the surface.
Most of the neoplastic cells are reasonably well-granulated and eosinophils are also present. There is
moderate variation in nuclear and cell size, with sometimes prominent nucleoli, some variation in
nuclear shape but no macro-, bi- or multi-nucleate mast cells seen. The mitotic count is 7 in 10 HPFs
(400×; 2.37 mm²).

   5   WHAT PATNAIK AND KIUPEL GRADING WOULD YOU ASSIGN TO THIS MCT?
       This mass is a Patnaik intermediate grade (grade II) and Kiupel high grade (for example, due to
       the mitotic count of 7).

Additional testing results:
   Ki67 = 18
   AgNOR = 3.1
   KIAG = 55.8
   KIT pattern 2
   Negative for *c-KIT* mutations (exon 7 and 11)

   6   ARE ANY OF THESE RESULTS OF CAUSE FOR CONCERN?
       KIAG is above the threshold, but only just (cut-off value is 54). KIT pattern II possibly of cause for
       concern, depending on the study you read!

Part II – canine soft tissue sarcoma (soft tissue tumours)

CASE 4

This case is an 8-year 9-month-old, male (neutered) crossbreed dog. Two masses are present, described
as subcutaneous in location; the first is a lipoma but the second mass is a STS.

Key features The mass is well-demarcated from the surrounding tissues, but has a mildly infiltrative growth pattern. The tumour cells are well-differentiated and spindle-shaped, with mild anisocytosis. There is no evidence of necrosis within the mass, although there are some perivascular lymphoid aggregates present. There is mild anisokaryosis with sometimes prominent nucleoli but no bi- or multi-nucleate cells. The mitotic count is 3 in 10 HPFs (400×; 2.37 mm^2).

7 WHAT HISTOLOGICAL GRADE WOULD YOU ASSIGN TO THIS SOFT TISSUE SARCOMA?
   Low grade (grade I).

CASE 5
This case is of a 9-year 7-month-old, male (neutered) Boxer. The clinical history is of a large mass on the cranial aspect of the left stifle. The mass is described as having tripled in size in 6 weeks.

Key features The mass is moderately well-demarcated from the surrounding tissues, but has a peripherally infiltrative growth pattern and varies in cellularity depending on the field examined. The tumour cells are well-differentiated and spindle-shaped, elongated to polygonal in shape, with small to moderate amounts of cytoplasm and moderate anisocytosis. There are some small focal areas of necrosis within the mass, and extensive inflammatory cell infiltrates. There is moderate anisokaryosis with sometimes prominent nucleoli. The mitotic count is 10 in 10 HPFs (400×; 2.37 mm^2).

8 WHAT HISTOLOGICAL GRADE WOULD YOU ASSIGN TO THIS SOFT TISSUE SARCOMA?
   Intermediate grade (grade II).

CASE 6
This case is of an 8-year 3-month-old, male (neutered) Springer spaniel dog. The clinical history is of a mass on the caudal aspect of the right hind limb.

Key features This mass is moderately cellular, unencapsulated, infiltrative and moderately well-demarcated from the surrounding tissues, and contains multifocal, often extensive areas of necrosis accounting for more than 50% of the tumour present in these sections. There is moderate anisocytosis, and moderate to marked anisokaryosis, with some multi-nucleate cells and a mitotic count of 32 in 10 HPFs (400×; 2.37 mm^2).

9 WHAT HISTOLOGICAL GRADE WOULD YOU ASSIGN TO THIS SOFT TISSUE SARCOMA?
   High grade (grade III).

References

Avallone, G., Rasotto, R., Chambers, J. K., et al. (2021) Review of histological grading systems in veterinary medicine. *Veterinary Pathology* 58(5): 809–828. https://doi.org/10.1177/0300985821999831.

Couto, S.S., Griffey, S.M., Duarte, P.C. & Madewell, B.R. (2002) Feline vaccine-associated fibrosarcoma: morphological distinctions. *Veterinary Pathology* 39: 33–41. https://doi.org/10.1354/vp.39-1-33.

Dagher, E., Abadie, J., Loussouarn, D. et al. (2019) Feline invasive mammary carcinomas: prognostic value of histological grading. *Veterinary Pathology* 56(5): 660–670. https://doi.org/10.1177/0300985819846870.

Davidson, G. A., Taylor, S. S., Dobromylskyj, M. J., Gemignani, F. & Renfrew, H. (2016) A case of an intramural, cavitated feline gastrointestinal eosinophilic sclerosing fibroplasia of the cranial abdomen in a domestic longhair cat. *Journal of Feline Medicine and Surgery Open Reports* 7(1). https://doi.org/10.1177/2055116921995396.

Dennis, M. M., McSporran, K. D., Bacon, N. J., Schulman, F. Y., Foster, R.A. & Powers, B. E. (2011) Prognostic factors for cutaneous and subcutaneous soft tissue sarcomas in dogs. *Veterinary Pathology* 48(1): 73–84. https://doi.org/10.1177/0300985810388820.

Dobromylskyj, M. J. & Little, C. J. (2021) Necropsy findings in a cat with diabetes mellitus and heart failure. *Journal of Feline Medicine and Surgery Open Reports* 7(2) https://doi.org/10.1177/20551169211055383.

Dobromylskyj, M. J., Copas, V., Durham, A., Hughes, T. K. & Patterson-Kane, J. C. (2011) Disseminated lipid-rich peritoneal mesothelioma in a horse. *Journal of Veterinary Diagnostic Investigation* 23(3): 615–618. https://doi.org/10.1177/1040638711403902.

Dobromylskyj, M. J., Rasotto, R., Melville, K., Smith, K. C. & Berlato, D. (2015) Evaluation of minichromosome Maintenance Protein 7 and c-KIT as prognostic markers in feline cutaneous mast cell tumours. *Journal of Comparative Pathology* 153(4): 244–250. https://doi.org/10.1016/j.jcpa.2015.08.005.

Dobromylskyj, M. J., Richards V. & Smith, K. C. (2021) Prognostic factors and proposed grading system for cutaneous and subcutaneous soft tissue sarcomas in cats, based on a retrospective study. *Journal of Feline Medicine and Surgery* 23(2): 168–174. https://doi.org/10.1177/1098612X20942393.

Kiupel, M., Webster, J. D., Bailey, K. L., et al. (2011) Proposal of a 2-tier histologic grading system for canine cutaneous mast cell tumors to more accurately predict biological behavior. *Veterinary Pathology* 48(1): 147–155. https://doi.org/10.1177/0300985810386469.

Koehler, J. W., Miller, A. D., Miller, C. R., et al. (2018) A revised diagnostic classification of canine glioma: towards validation of the canine glioma patient as a naturally occurring preclinical model for human glioma. *Journal of Neuropathology & Experimental Neurology* 77(11): 1039–1054. https://doi.org/10.1093/jnen/nly085.

Linden, D., Liptak, J. M., Vinayak, A., et al. (2019) Outcomes and prognostic variables associated with primary abdominal visceral soft tissue sarcomas in dogs: a veterinary society of surgical oncology retrospective study. *Veterinary and Comparative Oncology* 17: 265–270. https://doi.org/10.1111/vco.12456.

Luis Fuentes, V., Abbott, J., Chetboul, V., Côté, E., Fox, P. R., Häggström, J., Kittleson, M. D., Schober, K. & Stern, J. A. (2020) ACVIM consensus statement guidelines for the classification, diagnosis, and management of cardiomyopathies in cats. *Journal of Veterinary Internal Medicine* 34(3):1062–1077.

McSporran, K. D. (2009) Histologic grade predicts recurrence for marginally excised canine subcutaneous soft tissue sarcomas. *Veterinary Pathology* 46: 928–933. https://doi.org/10.1354/vp.08-VP-0277-M-FL.

Melville, K., Smith, K.C. & Dobromylskyj, M.J. (2015) Feline cutaneous mast cell tumours: a UK-based study comparing signalment and histological features with long-term outcomes. *Journal of Feline Medicine and Surgery* 17(6): 486–493. https://doi.org/10.1177/1098612X14548784.

Mills, S. W., Musil, K. M., Davies, J.L. et al. (2015) Prognostic value of histological grading for feline mammary carcinoma: a retrospective survival analysis. *Veterinary Pathology* 52(2): 238–249. https://doi.org/10.1177/0300985814543198.

Niessen, S. J. M., Voyce, M. J., De Villiers, L., Hargreaves, J., Blunden, A. S. & Syme, H. M. (2007) Generalised lymphadenomegaly associated with methimazole treatment in a hyperthyroid cat. *Journal of Small Animal Practice* 48: 165–168. https://doi.org/10.1111/j.1748-5827.2006.00186.x.

Porcellato, I., Menchetti, L., Brachelente, C. et al. (2017) Feline injection-site sarcoma: matrix remodeling and prognosis. *Veterinary Pathology* 54(2): 204–211. https://doi.org/10.1177/0300985816677148.

Sabattini, S. & Bettini, G. (2019) Grading cutaneous mast cell tumors in cats. *Veterinary Pathology* 56(1): 43–49. https://doi.org/10.1177/0300985818800028.

Sabattini, S., Guadagni Frizzon, M., Gentilini, F., Turba, M. E., Capitani, O. & Bettini, G. (2013) Prognostic significance of Kit receptor tyrosine kinase dysregulations in feline cutaneous mast cell tumors. *Veterinary Pathology* 50(5): 797–805. https://doi.org/10.1177/0300985813476064.

Smedley, R. C., Spangler, W. L., Esplin, D. G., Kitchell, B. E., Bergman, P. J., Ho, H. Y., Bergin, I. L. & Kiupel, M. (2011) Prognostic markers for canine melanocytic neoplasms: a comparative review of the literature and goals for future investigation. *Veterinary Pathology* 48(1): 54–72. https://doi.org/10.1177/0300985810390717.

Smedley, R. C., Bongiovanni, L., Bacmeister, C., Clifford, C.A., Christensen, N., Dreyfus, J.M., Gary, J.M., Pavuk, A., Rowland, P.H., Swanson, C., Tripp, C., Woods, J.P. & Bergman, P.J. (2022) Diagnosis and histopathologic prognostication of canine melanocytic neoplasms: a consensus of the Oncology-Pathology Working Group. *Veterinary and Comparative Oncology* 20(4): 739–751. https://doi.org/10.1111/vco.12827.

Trojani, M., Contesso, G., Coindre, J. M., Rouesse, J., Bui, N. B., De Mascarel, A., Goussot, J. F., David, M., Bonichon, F. & Lagarde, C. (1984) Soft-tissue sarcomas of adults; study of pathological prognostic variables and definition of a histopathological grading system. *International Journal of Cancer* 33: 37–42. https://doi.org/10.1002/ijc.2910330108.

Valli, V. E., Jacobs, A. L., Parodi, A. L. et al. (2002) Histological classification of hematopoietic tumors of domestic animals. In: Schulman, F.Y. (ed.) *World Health Organization International Histological Classification of Tumors of Domestic Animals*. Armed Force Institute of Pathology.

Valli, V. E., San Myint, M., Barthel, A, et al. (2011) Classification of canine malignant lymphomas according to the World Health Organization criteria. *Veterinary Pathology* 48(1): 198–211. https://doi.org/10.1177/0300985810379428.

Valli, V. E., Kass, P. H., San Myint, M. & Scott, F. (2013) Canine lymphomas: association of classification type, disease stage, tumor subtype, mitotic rate, and treatment with survival. *Veterinary Pathology* 50(5): 738–748. https://doi.org/10.1177/0300985813478210.

Webster, C. R. L., Center, S. A., Cullen, J. M., Penninck, D. G., Richter, K. P., Twedt, D. C. & Watson, P. J. (2019) ACVIM consensus statement on the diagnosis and treatment of chronic hepatitis in dogs. *Journal of Veterinary Internal Medicine* 33(3): 1173–1200. https://doi.org/10.1111/jvim.15467.

Further reading

Chapter 1 – Submission of samples

Stidworthy, M. & Priestnall, S. (2011) Getting the best results from veterinary histopathology. *In Practice* 33: 252–260. https://doi.org/10.1136/inp.d3598.

Chapter 2 – Post-mortem examinations and gross pathology

Dobromylskyj, M. J. & Little, C. J. (2021) Necropsy findings in a cat with diabetes mellitus and heart failure. *Journal of Feline Medicine and Surgery Open Reports* 7(2) https://doi.org/10.1177/20551169211055383.

King, J. M., Dodd, D. C. & Roth L. (2006) *The Necropsy Book: A Guide for Veterinary Students, Residents, Clinicians, Pathologists, and Biological Researchers*. Charles Lewis Davis Foundation.

Koehler, J. W., Miller, A. D., Miller, C. R., et al. (2018) A revised diagnostic classification of canine glioma: towards validation of the canine glioma patient as a naturally occurring preclinical model for human glioma. *Journal of Neuropathology & Experimental Neurology* 77(11): 1039–1054. https://doi.org/10.1093/jnen/nly085.

McDonough, S. P. & Southard, T. (2016) *Necropsy Guide for Dogs, Cats and Small Mammals*. Wiley Blackwell. https://doi.org/10.1002/9781119317005.

Moreland, R. E. (2009) *Color Atlas of Small Animal Necropsy*. Lulu.

Chapter 3 – Biopsy types with regards to tumour grading and margin assessment

Halsted, W. S. (1894) The results of operations for the cure of cancer of the breast performed at the John Hopkins Hospital from June 1889 to January 1894. *Annals of Surgery* 20(5): 497–555. https://doi.org/10.1097/00000658-189407000-00075.

Kamstock, D. A., Ehrhart, E.J., Getzy, D. M., et al. (2011) Recommended guidelines for submission, trimming, margin evaluation, and reporting of tumor biopsy specimens in veterinary surgical pathology. *Veterinary Pathology* 48(1): 19–31. https://doi.org/10.1177/0300985810389316.

Kiser, P. K., Löhr, C. V., Meritet, D., Spagnoli, S. T., Milovancev, M. & Russell, D. S. (2018) Histologic processing artifacts and inter-pathologist variation in measurement of inked margins of canine mast cell tumors. *Journal of Veterinary Diagnostic Investigation* 30(3): 377–385. https://doi.org/10.1177/1040638718757582.

Meuten, D. J., Moore, F. M., Donovan, T. A., et al. (2021) International guidelines for veterinary tumor pathology: a call to action. *Veterinary Pathology* 58(5): 766–794. https://doi.org/10.1177/03009858211013712.

Milovancev, M. & Russell, D. S. (2017) Surgical margins in the veterinary cancer patient. *Veterinary and Comparative Oncology* 15(4): 1136–1157. https://doi.org/10.1111/vco.12284.

Milovancev, M., Löhr, C. V., Bildfell, R. J., Gelberg, H. B., Heidel, J. R. & Valentine, B. A. (2013) A comparison of microscopic ink characteristics of 35 commercially available surgical margin inks. *Veterinary Surgery* 42(8): 901–908. https://doi.org/10.1111/j.1532-950X.2013.12069.x.

Roccobianca, P., Schulman, Y., Avallone, et al. (eds) (1974) *Surgical Pathology of Tumours of Domestic Animals. Volume 3: Tumours of Soft Tissue*. Davis-Thompson DVM Foundation.

Veterinary cancer guidelines and protocols – https://www.vcgp.org/.

Chapter 4 – Gastrointestinal and liver biopsies

Allenspach, K. A., Mochel, J. P., Du, Y., Priestnall, S. L., Moore, F., Slayter, M., Rodrigues, A., Ackermann, M., Krockenberger, M., Mansell, J., WSAVA GI Standardization Working Group, Luckschander, N., Wang, C., Suchodolski, J., Berghoff, N. & Jergens, A. E. (2019) Correlating gastrointestinal histopathologic changes to clinical disease activity in dogs with idiopathic inflammatory bowel disease. *Veterinary Pathology* 56(3): 435–443. https://doi.org/10.1177/0300985818813090.

Davidson, G. A., Taylor, S. S., Dobromylskyj, M. J., Gemignani, F. & Renfrew, H. (2016) A case of an intramural, cavitated feline gastrointestinal eosinophilic sclerosing fibroplasia of the cranial abdomen in a domestic longhair cat. *Journal of Feline Medicine and Surgery Open Reports* 7(1). https://doi.org/10.1177/2055116921995396.

Day, M. J., Bilzer, T., Mansell, J., Wilcock, B., Hall, E. J., Jergens, A., Minami, T., Willard, M., Washabau, R. & World Small Animal Veterinary Association Gastrointestinal Standardization Group (2008) Histopathological standards for the diagnosis of gastrointestinal inflammation in endoscopic biopsy samples from the dog and cat: a report from the World Small Animal Veterinary Association Gastrointestinal Standardization Group. *Journal of Comparative Pathology* 138(Suppl. 1): S1–43. https://doi.org/10.1016/j.jcpa.2008.01.001.

Dobromylskyj, M. J. (2016) Gastrointestinal biopsies from the pathologist's point of view. *Companion Animal Journal* 21(5). https://doi.org/10.12968/coan.2016.21.5.293.

Irving, J., Dobromylskyj, M. & Holmes, E. (2019) Feline alimentary lymphoma: a guide to cytological and histopathological diagnosis for the general practitioner. *Companion Animal Journal* 24(9). https://doi.org/10.12968/coan.2019.0033.

Johnson, G. F., Gilbertson, S. R., Goldfischer, S., Grushoff, P. S. & Sternlieb, I. (1984) Cytochemical detection of inherited copper toxicosis of bedlington terriers. *Veterinary Pathology* 21(1): 57–60. https://doi.org/10.1177/030098588402100110.

Kiupel, M., Smedley, R. C., Pfent, C., Xie, Y., Xue, Y., Wise, A. G., DeVaul, J. M. & Maes, R. K. (2011) Diagnostic algorithm to differentiate lymphoma from inflammation in feline small intestinal biopsy samples. *Veterinary Pathology* 48(1): 212–222. https://doi.org/10.1177/0300985810389479.

Moore, P. F., Rodriguez-Bertos, A. & Kass, P. H. (2012) Feline gastrointestinal lymphoma: mucosal architecture, immunophenotype, and molecular clonality. *Veterinary Pathology* 49(4): 658–668. https://doi.org/10.1177/0300985811404712.

Washabau, R. J., Day, M. J., Willard, M. D., Hall, E. J., Jergens, A. E., Mansell, J., Minami, T., Bilzer, T. W. & WSAVA International Gastrointestinal Standardization Group (2010) Endoscopic, biopsy, and histopathologic guidelines for the evaluation of gastrointestinal inflammation in companion animals. *Journal of Veterinary Internal Medicine* 24(1): 10–26. https://doi.org/10.1111/j.1939-1676.2009.0443.x.

Webster, C. R. L., Center, S. A., Cullen, J. M., Penninck, D. G., Richter, K. P., Twedt, D. C. & Watson, P. J. (2019) ACVIM consensus statement on the diagnosis and treatment of chronic hepatitis in dogs. *Journal of Veterinary Internal Medicine* 33(3): 1173–1200. https://doi.org/10.1111/jvim.15467.

Willard, M. & Mansell, J. (2011) Correlating clinical activity and histopathologic assessment of gastrointestinal lesion severity: current challenges. *Veterinary Clinics of North America. Small Animal Practice* 41(2): 457–463. https://doi.org/10.1016/j.cvsm.2011.01.005.

Chapter 5 – Special stains, immunohistochemistry and additional testing

Dobromylskyj, M. J. (2016) Using immunohistochemistry to help diagnose challenging tumours. *Companion Animal Journal* 21(12). https://doi.org/10.12968/coan.2016.21.12.702.

Dobromylskyj, M. J. (2016) What's so special about special stains? *Continuing Veterinary Education's Control & Therapy Series* 285.

Dobromylskyj, M. J., Copas, V., Durham, A., Hughes, T. K. & Patterson-Kane, J. C. (2011) Disseminated lipid-rich peritoneal mesothelioma in a horse. *Journal of Veterinary Diagnostic Investigation* 23(3): 615–618. https://doi.org/10.1177/1040638711403902.

Dobromylskyj, M. J., Rasotto, R., Melville, K., Smith, K. C. & Berlato, D. (2015) Evaluation of minichromosome Maintenance Protein 7 and c-KIT as prognostic markers in feline cutaneous mast cell tumours. *Journal of Comparative Pathology* 153(4): 244–250. https://doi.org/10.1016/j.jcpa.2015.08.005.

Priestnall, S. & Suárez-Bonnet, A. (2022) Additional stains and immunohistochemistry: what else can the pathologist tell us? *In Practice* 44(7): 385–393. https://doi.org/10.1002/inpr.90.

Chapter 6 – Oncology: recognising features of neoplasia and of malignancy

Niessen, S. J. M., Voyce, M. J., De Villiers, L., Hargreaves, J., Blunden, A. S. & Syme, H. M. (2007) Generalised lymphadenomegaly associated with methimazole treatment in a hyperthyroid cat. *Journal of Small Animal Practice* 48: 165–168. https://doi.org/10.1111/j.1748-5827.2006.00186.x.

Weishaar, K. M., Thamm, D. H., Worley, D. R. & Kamstock, D. A. (2014) Correlation of nodal mast cells with clinical outcome in dogs with mast cell tumour and a proposed classification system for the evaluation of node metastasis. *Journal of Comparative Pathology* 151(4): 329–338. https://doi.org/10.1016/j.jcpa.2014.07.004.

Chapter 7 – Oncology: histological descriptions, grading of neoplasms and additional prognostication

Overall review of histological grading systems

Avallone, G., Rasotto, R., Chambers, J. K., et al. (2021) Review of histological grading systems in veterinary medicine. *Veterinary Pathology* 58(5): 809–828. https://doi.org/10.1177/0300985821999831.

See also: Veterinary Cancer Guidelines and Protocols – https://www.vcgp.org/.

Canine MCTs

Bostock, D. E. (1973) The prognosis following surgical removal of mastocytomas in dogs. *Journal of Small Animal Practice* 14(1): 27–41. https://doi.org/10.1111/j.1748-5827.1973.tb06891.x.

Kiupel, M., Webster, J. D., Bailey, K. L., et al. (2011) Proposal of a 2-tier histologic grading system for canine cutaneous mast cell tumors to more accurately predict biological behavior. *Veterinary Pathology* 48(1): 147–155. https://doi.org/10.1177/0300985810386469.

Patnaik, A. K., Ehler, W. J. & MacEwen, E. G. (1984) Canine cutaneous mast cell tumour: morphological grading and survival time in 83 dogs. *Veterinary Pathology* 21(5): 469–474. https://doi.org/10.1177/030098588402100503.

Feline MCTs

Melville, K., Smith, K.C. & Dobromylskyj, M.J. (2015) Feline cutaneous mast cell tumours: a UK-based study comparing signalment and histological features with long-term outcomes. *Journal of Feline Medicine and Surgery* 17(6): 486–493. https://doi.org/10.1177/1098612X14548784.

Sabattini, S. & Bettini, G. (2019) Grading cutaneous mast cell tumors in cats. *Veterinary Pathology* 56(1): 43–49. https://doi.org/10.1177/0300985818800028.

Trojani, M., Contesso, G., Coindre, J. M., Rouesse, J., Bui, N. B., De Mascarel, A., Goussot, J. F., David, M., Bonichon, F. & Lagarde, C. (1984) Soft-tissue sarcomas of adults; study of pathological prognostic variables and definition of a histopathological grading system. *International Journal of Cancer* 33: 37–42. https://doi.org/10.1002/ijc.2910330108.

Canine STS

David, M., Bonichon, F. & Lagarde, C. (1984) Soft-tissue sarcomas of adults; study of pathological prognostic variables and definition of a histopathological grading system. *International Journal of Cancer* 33: 37–42. https://doi.org/10.1002/ijc.2910330108.

Dennis, M. M., McSporran, K. D., Bacon, N. J., Schulman, F. Y., Foster, R.A. & Powers, B. E. (2011) Prognostic factors for cutaneous and subcutaneous soft tissue sarcomas in dogs. *Veterinary Pathology* 48(1): 73–84. https://doi.org/10.1177/0300985810388820.

Linden, D., Liptak, J. M., Vinayak, A., et al. (2019) Outcomes and prognostic variables associated with primary abdominal visceral soft tissue sarcomas in dogs: a veterinary society of surgical oncology retrospective study. *Veterinary and Comparative Oncology* 17: 265–270. https://doi.org/10.1111/vco.12456.

McSporran, K. D. (2009) Histologic grade predicts recurrence for marginally excised canine subcutaneous soft tissue sarcomas. *Veterinary Pathology* 46: 928–933. https://doi.org/10.1354/vp.08-VP-0277-M-FL.

Feline STS

Couto, S.S., Griffey, S.M., Duarte, P.C. & Madewell, B.R. (2002) Feline vaccine-associated fibrosarcoma: morphological distinctions. *Veterinary Pathology* 39: 33–41. https://doi.org/10.1354/vp.39-1-33.

Dobromylskyj, M. J., Richards V. & Smith, K. C. (2021) Prognostic factors and proposed grading system for cutaneous and subcutaneous soft tissue sarcomas in cats, based on a retrospective study. *Journal of Feline Medicine and Surgery* 23(2): 168–174. https://doi.org/10.1177/1098612X20942393.

Porcellato, I., Menchetti, L., Brachelente, C. et al. (2017) Feline injection-site sarcoma: matrix remodeling and prognosis. *Veterinary Pathology* 54(2): 204–211. https://doi.org/10.1177/0300985816677148.

Lymphoma

Valli, V. E., Jacobs, A. L., Parodi, A. L. et al. (2002) Histological classification of hematopoietic tumors of domestic animals. In: Schulman, F.Y. (ed.) *World Health Organization International Histological Classification of Tumors of Domestic Animals*. Armed Force Institute of Pathology.

Valli, V. E., Kass, P. H., San Myint, M. & Scott, F. (2013) Canine lymphomas: association of classification type, disease stage, tumor subtype, mitotic rate, and treatment with survival. *Veterinary Pathology* 50(5): 738–748. https://doi.org/10.1177/0300985813478210.

Valli, V. E., San Myint, M., Barthel, A, et al. (2011) Classification of canine malignant lymphomas according to the World Health Organization criteria. *Veterinary Pathology* 48(1): 198–211. https://doi.org/10.1177/0300985810379428.

Canine mammary carcinoma

Peña, L., De Andres, P. J. D., Clemente, M. et al. (2013) Prognostic value of histological grading in non-inflammatory canine mammary carcinomas in a prospective study with two-year follow-up: relationship with clinical and histological characteristics. *Veterinary Pathology* 50(1): 94–105. https://doi.org/10.1177/0300985812447830.

Feline mammary carcinoma

Dagher, E., Abadie, J., Loussouarn, D. et al. (2019) Feline invasive mammary carcinomas: prognostic value of histological grading. *Veterinary Pathology* 56(5): 660–670. https://doi.org/10.1177/0300985819846870.

Mills, S. W., Musil, K. M., Davies, J .L. et al. (2015) Prognostic value of histological grading for feline mammary carcinoma: a retrospective survival analysis. *Veterinary Pathology* 52(2): 238–249. https://doi.org/10.1177/0300985814543198.

Canine pulmonary carcinoma

McNiel, E. A., Ogilvie, G. K., Powers, B. E. et al. (1997) Evaluation of prognostic factors for dogs with primary lung tumours: 67 cases (1985–1992). *Journal of the American Veterinary Medical Association* 211(11): 1422–1427.

Additional prognostic testing

Canine MCTs

Abadie, J. J., Amardeilh, M. A. & Delverdier, M. E. (1999) Immunohistochemical detection of proliferating cell nuclear antigen and Ki-67 in mast cell tumors from dogs. *Journal of the American Veterinary Medical Association* 215(11): 1629–1634.

Bostock, D. E., Crocker, J., Harris, K., & Smith, P. (1989) Nucleolar organiser regions as indicators of post-surgical prognosis in canine spontaneous mast cell tumours. *British Journal of Cancer* 59(6): 915–918. https://doi.org/10.1038/bjc.1989.193.

Giantin, M., Vascellari, M., Morello, E. M., Capello, K., Vercelli, A., Granato, A., Lopparelli, R. M., Nassuato, C., Carminato, A., Martano, M., Mutinelli, F. & Dacasto, M. (2012) c-KIT messenger RNA and protein expression and mutations in canine cutaneous mast cell tumors: correlations with post-surgical prognosis. *Journal of Veterinary Diagnostic Investigation* 24(1): 116–126. https://doi.org/10.1177/1040638711425945.

Kiupel, M., Webster, J. D., Kaneene, J. B., Miller, R. & Yuzbasiyan-Gurkan, V. (2004) The use of KIT and tryptase expression patterns as prognostic tools for canine cutaneous mast cell tumors. *Veterinary Pathology* 41(4): 371–377. https://doi.org/10.1354/vp.41-4-371.

Maglennon, G. A., Murphy, S., Adams, V., Miller, J., Smith, K., Blunden, A. & Scase, T. J. (2008) Association of Ki67 index with prognosis for intermediate-grade canine cutaneous mast cell tumours. *Veterinary and Comparative Oncology* 6(4): 268–274. https://doi.org/10.1111/j.1476-5829.2008.00168.x.

Newman, S. J., Mrkonjich, L., Walker, K. K. & Rohrbach, B. W. (2007) Canine subcutaneous mast cell tumour: diagnosis and prognosis. *Journal of Comparative Pathology* 136(4): 231–239. https://doi.org/10.1016/j.jcpa.2007.02.003.

Scase, T. J., Edwards, D., Miller, J., Henley, W., Smith, K., Blunden, A. & Murphy, S. (2006) Canine mast cell tumors: Correlation of apoptosis and proliferation markers with prognosis. *Journal of Veterinary Internal Medicine* 20(1): 151–158. https://doi.org/10.1111/j.1939-1676.2006.tb02835.x.

Simoes, J. P., Schoning, P. & Butine, M. (1994) Prognosis of canine mast cell tumors: a comparison of three methods. *Veterinary Pathology* 31(6): 637–647. https://doi.org/10.1177/030098589403100602.

Thompson, J. J., Pearl, D. L., Yager, J. A., Best, S. J., Coomber, B. L., & Foster, R. A. (2011) Canine subcutaneous mast cell tumor: Characterization and prognostic indices. *Veterinary Pathology*, 48(1): 156–168. https://doi.org/10.1177/0300985810387446.

Thompson, J. J., Yager, J. A., Best, S. J., Pearl, D. L., Coomber, B. L., Torres, R. N., Kiupel, M. & Foster, R. A. (2011) Canine subcutaneous mast cell tumors: cellular proliferation and KIT expression as prognostic indices. *Veterinary Pathology* 48(1): 169–181. https://doi.org/10.1177/0300985810390716.

Webster, J. D., Yuzbasiyan-Gurkan, V., Miller, R. A., Kaneene, J. B. & Kiupel, M. (2007) Cellular proliferation in canine cutaneous mast cell tumors: associations with c-KIT and its role in prognostication. *Veterinary Pathology* 44(3): 298–308. https://doi.org/10.1354/vp.44-3-298.

Webster, J. D., Yuzbasiyan-Gurkan, V., Thamm, D. H., Hamilton, E. & Kiupel, M. (2008) Evaluation of prognostic markers for canine mast cell tumors treated with vinblastine and prednisone. *BMC Veterinary Research* 4, 32. https://doi.org/10.1186/1746-6148-4-32.

Zemke, D., Yamini, B. & Yuzbasiyan-Gurkan, V. (2002) Mutations in the juxtamembrane domain of c-KIT are associated with higher grade mast cell tumors in dogs. *Veterinary Pathology* 39(5): 529–535. https://doi.org/10.1354/vp.39-5-529.

Feline MCTs

Dobromylskyj, M. J., Rasotto, R., Melville, K., Smith, K. C. & Berlato, D. (2015) Evaluation of minichromosome maintenance Protein 7 and c-KIT as prognostic markers in feline cutaneous mast cell tumours. *Journal of Comparative Pathology* 153(4): 244–250. https://doi.org/10.1016/j.jcpa.2015.08.005.

Sabattini, S. & Bettini, G. (2010) Prognostic value of histologic and immunohistochemical features in feline cutaneous mast cell tumors. *Veterinary Pathology* 47(4): 643–653. https://doi.org/10.1177/0300985810364509.

Sabattini, S., Guadagni Frizzon, M., Gentilini, F., Turba, M. E., Capitani, O. & Bettini, G. (2013) Prognostic significance of Kit receptor tyrosine kinase dysregulations in feline cutaneous mast cell tumors. *Veterinary Pathology* 50(5): 797–805. https://doi.org/10.1177/0300985813476064.

Canine melanocytic neoplasms

Smedley, R. C., Bongiovanni, L., Bacmeister, C., Clifford, C.A., Christensen, N., Dreyfus, J.M., Gary, J.M., Pavuk, A., Rowland, P.H., Swanson, C., Tripp, C., Woods, J.P. & Bergman, P.J. (2022) Diagnosis and histopathologic prognostication of canine melanocytic neoplasms: a consensus of the Oncology-Pathology Working Group. *Veterinary and Comparative Oncolology* 20(4): 739–751. https://doi.org/10.1111/vco.12827.

Smedley, R. C., Spangler, W. L., Esplin, D. G., Kitchell, B. E., Bergman, P. J., Ho, H. Y., Bergin, I. L. & Kiupel, M. (2011) Prognostic markers for canine melanocytic neoplasms: a comparative review of the literature and goals for future investigation. *Veterinary Pathology* 48(1): 54–72. https://doi.org/10.1177/0300985810390717.

Index

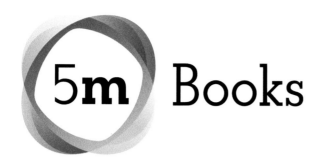

£100 FREE BOOKS?

Tell us about how you came to this book and we'll enter you in our next draw to win £100 of our books.

Scan the QR code to start or visit
https://forms.office.com/e/97P5QTyZmk

We at 5m are passionate about improving the health and happiness of the animals we farm and live with and of the environment we farm in.

Our mission is to publish the highest quality books in veterinary and animal sciences, agriculture and aquaculture.

Join us at www.5mbooks.com or follow our social media channels to be part of our community and to find out more about our books and authors.

We welcome proposals for new books in the areas in which we publish. We would be delighted to hear from you, please email us: hello@5mbooks.com

www.5mbooks.com

 @5mBooks | @5m_Books | @5m_Books
 linkedin.com/company/5mbooks